Abortion, Fertility, and Changing Legislation: An International Review

Abortion, Fertility, and Changing Legislation: An International Review

Jean van der Tak
Transnational Family Research Institute
American Institutes for Research
Washington, D.C.

Lexington Books
D.C. Heath and Company
Lexington, Massachusetts
Toronto London

Library of Congress Cataloging in Publication Data

Van der Tak, Jean.
Abortion, fertility, and changing legislation: an international review

Bibliography: p.
1. Abortion. 2. Fertility, Human. 3. Birth control. I. Title. [DNLM: 1. Abortion, Induced. 2. Abortion, Legal. 3. Fertility. HQ767 V231a 1974]
HQ76.V36 301.32'1 74-4023
ISBN 0-669-94029-1

Published simultaneously in Canada.

Printed in the United States of America.

International Standard Book Number: 0-669-94029-1

Library of Congress Catalog Card Number: 74-4023

Contents

List of Figures

List of Tables

Foreword

Today's central problem of demographic analysis in the abortion field is essentially this: to derive from two sets of data quantitative estimates of three types of reproductive behavior. The two sets of data are the numbers and rates of live births and of legal abortions and the changes over time in these numbers and rates; the three types of human behavior are (1) replacement of illegal abortions by legal abortions; (2) replacement of live births by abortion, and (3) replacement of contraception (or avoidance of premarital coitus) by abortion. Owing to the private and covert nature of the behavior involved in these replacements, relevant information tends to be fragmentary, inferential, or nonexistent. Under these circumstances, more often than not, evidence is persuasive rather than conclusive. Ms. van der Tak's monograph represents the first attempt to review, consolidate, and interpret on a worldwide basis the findings of many workers in the expanding field of abortion research. I salute her courage, determination, and sound judgment in exploring this uncharted sea.

Christopher Tietze
The Population Council

Preface

Much has been said and written about abortion but the available facts are few. Long mired in a swamp of illegality and social ambivalence in large parts of the world, it has been difficult to organize and conduct systematic studies assessing the incidence of abortion and its role within the total context of human fertility regulating behavior. Jean van der Tak has now assembled available published and unpublished evidence from Europe, Asia, and North and South America to illustrate recent fertility trends associated with varying levels of induced abortion and contraception prevailing under different official abortion policies, legislation, and practice in diverse sociocultural milieus. The Transnational Family Research Institute and its associated International Reference Center for Abortion Research are proud to offer this unique contribution as the first of several planned publications.

This monograph was commissioned in the belief that an understanding of the complex interrelationships between abortion practices and fertility amidst changing legislative and enforcement conditions, as well as differing sociocultural milieus and expanding availability of modern contraception, would be of utility to policymakers, administrators, clinicians, researchers, family planning workers, and all others interested in assessing the abortion phenomenon in their own local, national, and regional contexts. While there have been previous attempts in selected situations to assess the effect on fertility of induced abortion, whether legal or illegal, integrative efforts have usually floundered amidst the admitted difficulties of collecting unassailable data with which to isolate the impact of abortion from that of numerous other factors likely to influence fertility trends, particularly concurrent changes in contraceptive practice and socioeconomic development. Probably for the same reason there have been few (if any) attempts to offer international comparisons, such as between developed and developing countries, or between societies with varying histories of contraceptive distribution, availability and practice. How then to assess the impact of abortion on unwanted fertility particularly when liberalization of abortion statutes might be under consideration?

While recognizing the softness of some of the data and the limitations of her approach, Jean van der Tak makes a convincing case for her finding that a voluntary reduction in birth rates—providing that the motivation for fertility regulation exists—is most likely to occur when both modern contraception and induced abortion, legal or condoned, are widely available. This conclusion dovetails with the public health and civil rights arguments for liberalizing abortion legislation and permitting women to decide whether or not to terminate an unwanted pregnancy (within specified time periods). It appears that reductions in fertility and improved contraceptive practice tend to be associated with initial increases in legal abortion and declines in highly dangerous illegal abortion, and also with a decrease in out-of-wedlock births and postponement of marriage, which potentially lowers completed fertility. The impression is persuasive that abortion deserves a place in family planning programs, adding "hindsight" capability to preventive endeavors. Within such a total approach it is quite likely, as has already been demonstrated in several countries, that the incidence of induced abortion will gradually level off while effective contraceptive practice increases and becomes the mainstay for attaining societally desired population growth rates.

While Jean van der Tak consulted with other members of the Transnational Family Research Institute and with our Technical Advisory Board, the monograph is entirely her own effort, produced with energy and dedication. We will be much interested in the views of others, as well as abortion studies that may have been inadvertently missed.

We hope that this and future publications will assist the worldwide effort to understand the reality of induced abortion and to separate fact from emotion.

Henry P. David
Director, Transnational Family
Research Institute

Acknowledgments

Resources for this review were drawn entirely from material collected by the International Reference Center for Abortion Research (IRCAR), established in 1971 by the Transnational Family Research Institute (TFRI). Special consultants for the report were Dr. Christopher Tietze of The Population Council, New York, and Dr. Malcolm Potts of the International Planned Parenthood Federation, London, both members of the IRCAR/TFRI Technical Advisory Board, who gave generously of their time and expertise. Their own extensive publications in the fields of abortion and contraception were indispensable sources of information and guidance, as was the *Inventory of Information on Induced Abortion* by Dr. Emily C. Moore-Cavar of the International Institute for the Study of Human Reproduction, Columbia University, which the author kindly made available in manuscript form. Dr. Henry P. David, Director of TFRI, inspired the original project and guided its development. Other colleagues who helped expertly in the preparation of the final manuscript were Adele E. Gunn, Mary G. Kalis, Dr. Patricia McCormick, Charles A. Poore, Ann G. Rosendall, and Marylis Sevilla-Que.

The Transnational Family Research Institute is a multidisciplinary nongovernmental, and nonprofit research organization, affiliated with the American Institutes for Research in the Behavioral Sciences, Washington, D.C. The following serve on the Technical Advisory Board:

Prof. Berislav Beric (Novi Sad, Yugoslavia)
Prof. Jean M. Kellerhals (Geneva, Switzerland)
Dr. Malcolm Potts (London, England)
Dr. Christopher Tietze (New York, N.Y., U.S.A.)

Abortion, Fertility, and Changing Legislation: An International Review

1 Introduction

With great sincerity, but some degree of inaccuracy, those interested in family planning have suggested that contraception alone will control human fertility to meet individual and communal goals and that contraception is a way of reducing illegal abortion rates. The situation is more complex. In broad terms, two generalizations seem possible: namely, that no developed country has achieved a decline in its birth rate without a considerable recourse to abortion—whether legal or illegal—and, secondly, that no developing country will achieve its target degree of fertility control without a considerable recourse to abortion—whether legal or illegal. (Potts, 177, pp. 11-12)

This book aims to present in summary, nontechnical fashion available evidence to document the above statement. It further seeks to illustrate that, to varying degrees, depending upon de facto liberalization and the nature and extent of concurrent contraceptive practice, legalization facilitates the most effective integration of abortion with contraception in an optimal combination of fertility-regulating methods which can be expected to have maximum impact on fertility trends. Berelson has suggested that "making induced abortions legal and illegal may be one of the most effective single ways the modern state has of changing birth rates up and down, although the Romanian case shows that its effect upward is not lasting" (16, p. 16).

Clearly, no government wishes to advocate abortion as a substitute for effective contraception in the attempt to reduce rates of population growth. However, a summary guide to the contribution legalization of abortion might make to this effort should be useful to decision makers in less developed countries where organized family planning programs have, to date, generally had little measurable impact on such growth (15, 129, 137, 157, 183), as well as those in developed countries where it is postulated that the elimination of unwanted or untimely births (due to faulty or nonuse of contraception) could reduce growth rates to near replacement levels (228).

The book does not deal with the heretofore main stated arguments for liberalization of restrictive abortion laws: that, as abortion has been and is universally practiced despite prohibitions, legalization will facilitate early, nondiscriminatory access to abortion under safe medical conditions, thus dramatically lowering the rates of maternal mortality and morbidity associated with illegal abortion, with their concomitant high societal and personal costs; and that legalization of abortion ensures to women the fundamental right to complete control of their own fertility. An abundant literature exists on these two topics.

Factors Involved in Assessing the Impact of Abortion on Fertility

To attempt to isolate abortion's impact on observed fertility trends involves consideration of the many other factors that influence such trends. Many of the relevant data are elusive and nonquantifiable, which probably explains the relative lack of professional attention to this issue to date. However, there is general agreement that the following factors must be taken into account in such an assessment, and it is against this background that this body of evidence is presented.

Relationship of Abortion and Contraception

Requena and Klinger have proposed a model that illustrates *three stages through which nations and social classes may pass in the demographic transition* from high to low rates of fertility (and mortality), from no birth prevention and high birth rates, to falling birth rates accomplished primarily by abortion, to low birth rates achieved mainly by contraception with some residual abortions to meet contraceptive failure (122, 187). Figure 1-1 shows stages over time as well as concurrent patterns observed in different strata of society at one point in time.

Some researchers argue that societies tend to move through these stages regardless of the legal status of abortion; e.g., that Japan's legalization of abortion in 1948 happened to coincide with that country's inevitable shift to Stage 2 in the model, while liberalization of abortion in Great Britain in 1967 "came a hundred years too late," after the inevitable bulge of abortions had subsided (along with thousands of unnecessary deaths) and the country's demographic transition had been largely accomplished (176).

Tietze and Dawson point out that induced abortion and contraception share a common objective: the prevention of unwanted births (231, p. 5). Therefore, *when societies and individuals are motivated to begin the effort to control their fertility abortion and contraceptive use can rise simultaneously.* If contraception fails or the demand exceeds supply (66), women thus motivated will resort to abortion to terminate unwanted or untimely pregnancies that they now find unacceptable. Similarly, women who have had abortions are more likely to use contraception than other women less motivated to control fertility (146, Chapter 10; 166; 231, p. 5). Thus, abortion and contraception are complementary rather than competitive means to control fertility (176). Over time, abortion is used increasingly to compensate for contraceptive failure, rather than as the primary method to limit births; hence it accounts for less substitution

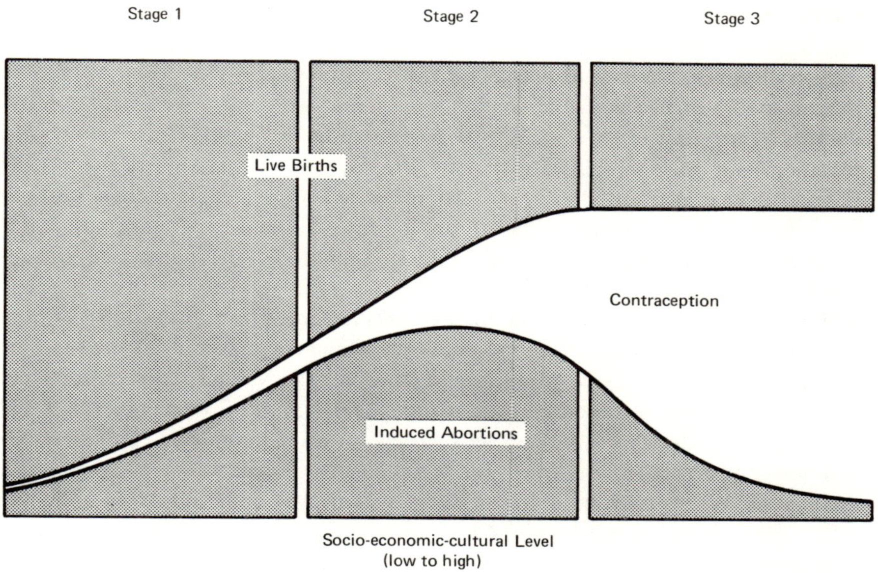

Figure 1-1. Historical and Social Stages of the Interrelationship of Live Births, Contraceptive Practice, and Induced Abortion. Source: Reprinted with permission of The Population Council from J.A. Ross, A. Germain, J.E. Forrest, and J. van Ginneken. Findings from family planning research, *Reports on Population/Family Planning*, No. 12 (October 1972), figure 2, p. 36.

effect and more net births prevented (195, p. 37). However, a substantial proportion of women may remain who find it easier to apply the "curative" method of abortion to deal with the certainty of a recognized pregnancy than adopt "preventive" contraceptive methods to deal with the (remote) possibility of conception (66, p. 130; 145, p. 133). It is uncertain how much of this attitude can be attributed to the high psychological costs of obtaining contraceptives for some women, especially the young and/or unmarried. Some observers have suggested that ready availability of abortion may encourage relaxation of contraceptive effort (145, pp. 139-40) or retard adoption of modern contraceptive methods, such as intrauterine devices (IUDs) or the pill (221).

Hulka has shown that *theoretically all presently available methods of reversible contraception are not sufficiently predictable to keep lifetime family size within the two or three children ideal* now almost universal within industrialized countries and hoped for in developing countries, if failures due to human errors in use and due to method defects are considered (101). Of 100 couples marrying in their early twenties, over 80 would have unplanned pregnancies in their remaining twelve to fifteen years of fertile marriage after the last desired conception if they consistently used 95 percent effective methods (such as the diaphragm or condom), and about 30 would experience unplanned pregnancies while using 99 percent effective methods (the IUD, according to some measurements, and the pill).

Potter has demonstrated that, *theoretically 100 abortions prevent fewer than 100 live births* (174). The interval between pregnancies consists of (1) the time taken to conceive, (2) the duration of the pregnancy, and (3) an interval of relative infertility. In the case of abortion, the duration of pregnancy is less and the return of fertility more rapid—especially when compared to pregnancy followed by breast-feeding—but the first factor, the time taken to conceive, is unchanged. Where only induced abortion is used, 100 abortions will avert only 30-43 births (i.e., it takes about two to three abortions to avert one birth), depending upon the duration of breast-feeding, and the number of conceptions (births plus abortions) will increase. Contraception lengthens (1), the time taken to conceive. Therefore, in a population using contraception, 100 abortions will avert up to 89 births (or, about 1.2 abortions = 1 averted birth), depending mainly upon contraceptive efficiency and, under certain conditions, upon age when birth control starts, and the number of conceptions decreases. This model "makes the point that abortion alone is an inefficient method of fertility regulation, becoming progressively more efficient as the expanding use of contraception relegates its role to a backstop measure" (Tietze and Dawson, 231, p. 6).

Using this approach, Venkatacharya has estimated that in India, if abortion were used as the sole means of fertility control, about 5.8 to 9.8 million induced abortions would have been required annually to reduce that country's birth rate 11 to 15 percent between 1960 and 1975 (254). In 1966, a government abortion review committee estimated that at least 4 million illegal abortions occurred annually in India (104). Despite de jure legalization in 1972 (see Chapter 2), the total has undoubtedly risen. Current estimates of birth rates and total population indicate that numbers of annual births in India now range between 21.4 and 25 million (107, 240).

Legal-Illegal Substitution

Legalization of abortion precipitates or accelerates declining trends in fertility only to the extent that it averts births that otherwise would occur. No net savings in births are effected when legal abortions merely substitute for what would have been illegal or "medical" abortions under earlier, more repressive abortion laws, or when it applies to "excess" pregnancies caused by legalization itself, such as those due to the increased numbers of women able to conceive again because their pregnancies were terminated by abortion, or those possibly due to relaxation of contraceptive effort or increased coital frequency in response to easier access to abortion (229). Estimation of the demographic impact of abortion legalization in this respect is complicated by the impossibility of ascertaining with accuracy the level of illegal abortion before legalization, and what this level might later have been in the absence of legalization (175). Because of its clandestine nature, the extent of illegal abortion can only be estimated by means of "informed" guesses, numbers of deaths attributed to abortion, hospital data on numbers of patients admitted for treatment of "incomplete" abortions—a certain percentage of which are assumed to be induced rather than spontaneous—and surveys that seek to elicit from women of childbearing age the percentage who have ever resorted to abortion (146, Chapter 6). (The World Health Organization estimates that spontaneous abortions terminate 15 to 20 percent of all pregnancies [268]. An abortion/pregnancy ratio in excess of this can be attributed to induced abortion. Diggory estimates that, in the conditions prevailing in Great Britain just before the 1967 Abortion Act, about one in five illegal abortions required subsequent hospitalization [66, 67].) Even where abortion has been legal for some time, as in Eastern Europe and Japan, such surveys are prone to underestimation of the proportion ever having had an abortion by perhaps as much as 30 to 50 percent (2, 151). By early 1973 official statistics on abortion were available from only 18 to 20 countries where abortion had been liberalized and for a variety of reasons even these are not considered reliable in all cases (58; 240: 1971, Table 25).

Abortion Used to Avert Timing Versus Number Failures

The impact of abortion on fertility trends also depends, as Bumpass and Presser point out, on the "extent to which aborted pregnancies would have resulted in births that were not wanted until later (timing failures) or in births that were not wanted at all (number failures). Family size clearly is reduced by abortion of pregnancies that are number failures" (29, p. 44). The majority of aborters in most countries tend to be married women (including the consensually mated, as in Latin America), aged 20 to 39 (231, Tables 4, 9), anxious to terminate such number failures after attainment of desired family size (two to three children in developed countries and three to five in less developed countries. See Appendix Table). However, there is evidence that *increasingly women under age 20, the unmarried, and women with no previous births*, confronted with unplanned pregnancies, *are resorting to abortion to avoid out-of-wedlock births and/or postpone first births*–i.e., timing failures. To the extent that legalization of abortion facilitates this trend, this might be the avenue of its greatest long-run impact on population growth. The postponement of first births inevitably alters the timing of births. This in turn lengthens the generation span and increases the likelihood of lower completed family size, since fecundity diminishes with age and once motherhood has been postponed, family size goals may well be revised downward. This reduces the potential size and growth of population in the future as well as current annual fertility rates (29, 34, 138, 228).

Analyzing data from a national sample of 17,000 U.S. women interviewed in 1967, half of whose first births occurred on average about 1947, Cutright and Galle estimate that eliminating first births conceived out of wedlock (13 percent of white and 52 percent of nonwhite first births among ever married women in the sample) would have reduced the completed fertility of these women only minimally–1.2 percent among whites and 2.6 percent among nonwhites. They also question the assumption that, up to 1968 in the United States at least, eliminating births conceived out of wedlock would substantially raise the mean age of mothers at childbearing, i.e., lengthen the generation span and thus slow population growth rates. However, these researchers also show that the 1968 U.S. general fertility rate of 84.4 births[a] per 1000 women aged 15 to 44 was inflated about 6.5 percent because of rising rates of out-of-wedlock childbearing after 1940, and note that 30 percent of wives under 25 interviewed nationally by the Census Bureau in June 1972 were pregnant at marriage (50). Evidence presented in this monograph from areas in the United States where legal abortion became widely available after 1967 suggests that broad liberalization of abortion on a national scale, as authorized by the U.S. Supreme Court decree of January 1973, should help dampen what otherwise would have been an increasing net impact of extramaritally conceived births on U.S. rates of population growth. This also appears to be true in Britain.

Abortion Rates and Ratios

A clear distinction should be made between abortion *rates* per 1000 population or per 1000 women, and abortion *ratios* per 1000 live births or pregnancies (abortions plus live births) (86; 145, pp. 137-38; 231, p. 5). A population or subpopulation with a relatively low birth rate due to successful use of contraception or exposure to low risks of conception because of infrequent sexual intercourse (very young and/or unmarried, divorced, separated, or widowed women) or declining fecundity (older women) may have a very low abortion *rate* but a very high abortion *ratio*. That is, unplanned pregnancies

[a]The final official report sets the general fertility rate of 1968 at 85.7 (250).

occur relatively infrequently, but once they do, they are very likely to be aborted.

De Facto Versus De Jure Status of Abortion

The degree to which legalization of abortion averts births that otherwise would occur is also dependent upon *the degree to which the law is liberalized in theory and in practice and services are available to meet the demand.* By January 1974, abortion at the unconditional request of any woman in the first three months of pregnancy was legally available in only seven countries: the People's Republic of China, Denmark, the German Democratic Republic, Tunisia, the U.S.S.R., the Democratic Republic of Vietnam, and the United States. In some twenty other countries elective abortion was legally available to certain categories of women: those of a certain age, marital status or parity, or whose abortions could be justified for socioeconomic or for broadly defined physical and mental health reasons. In all other countries abortion was technically illegal without exception, or permitted only under such restricted circumstances as rape, incest, or risk of a deformed fetus or serious danger to the pregnant woman's health or life (57). Figure 1-2 depicts the worldwide legal status of abortion as of January 1974, according to these three classifications. (It is estimated that as of this date more than half the world's population lives in the twenty-seven countries where abortion is legally available either on request during the first three months of pregnancy or on the broad terms of the second category [131].)

Despite relatively liberal laws, access to legal abortion remained difficult in Scandinavia before 1965, because of rigorous legal interpretation and laborious administrative practices, and in the United States and Great Britain in some areas, following recent legal changes, because of residual medical and societal opposition, and, in some cases, lack of facilities to meet the demand. On the other hand, despite legal restrictions, abortion performed by qualified medical personnel is apparently widely available in, among others, Israel, some cantons of Switzerland, Greece, The Netherlands, Taiwan, and the Republic of Korea. The impression prevails that this is true also for at least the affluent in most of Latin America and the Arab countries of the Near East.

An initial problem for less developed countries if they were to liberalize abortion (as in India in 1972 and Tunisia in 1973) *would be their ability to meet the resultant demand with adequate medical facilities* (181, p. 587). Safe, easily adaptable techniques, such as vacuum aspiration in the first trimester of pregnancy, administered on an outpatient basis, could substantially reduce the need for any elaborate medical infrastructure, as in the People's Republic of China, for instance, where, according to at least one recent report, the majority of abortions in cities are performed by nurses, and in rural areas by "barefoot doctors" (paramedical personnel) or midwives (72).

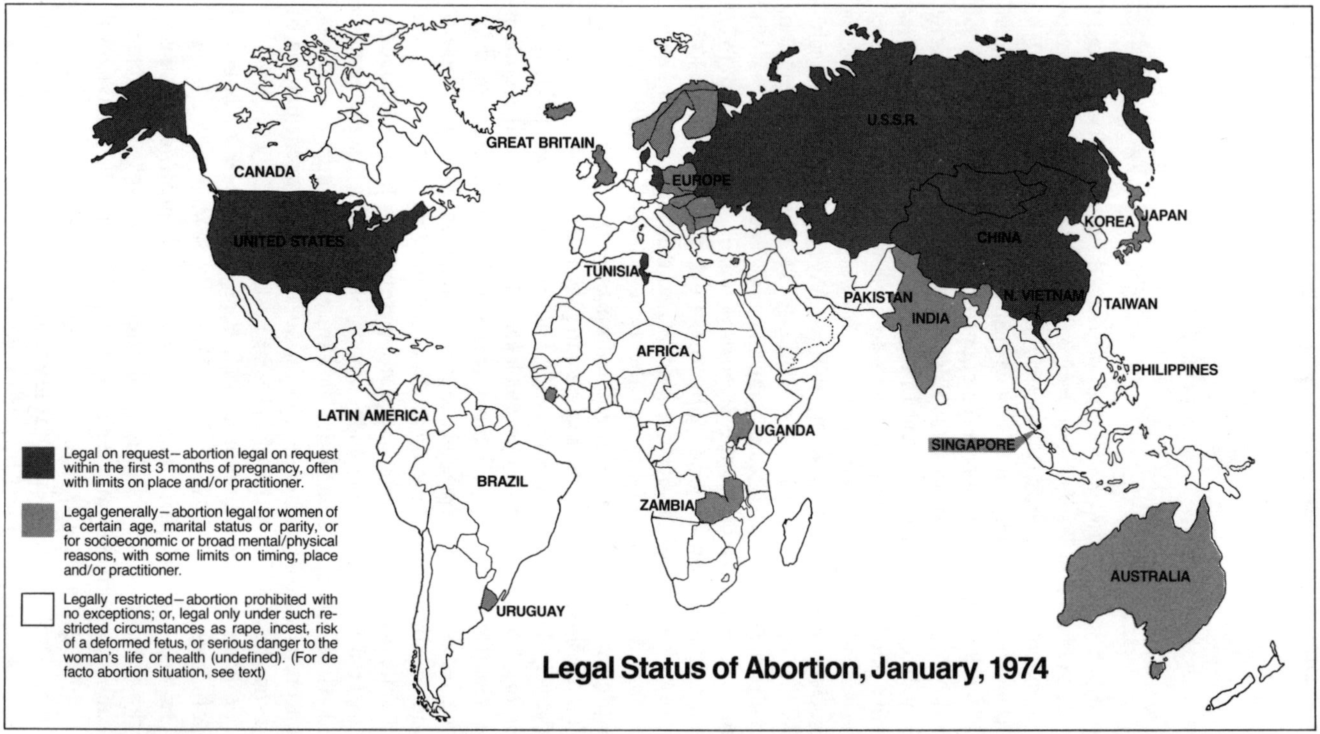

Figure 1-2. Legal Status of Abortion, January 1974. Source: Modified and updated from map appearing originally in L.T. Lee, Five largest countries allow legal abortion on broad grounds. *Population Report*, April 1973, Series F, No. 1. The original map was prepared by the Population Information Program in cooperation with IRCAR.

Other Factors Influencing Observed Fertility Trends

In general, abortion and contraception provide only the *means* to achieving lower levels of fertility. The *motivation* for smaller family sizes in the course of a country's demographic transition is usually stimulated by a variety of other factors.[b] "The list could be long, little is known about the relative importance of each factor and a suitable way of measuring the quantitative impact of a given factor is lacking" (152, p. 90). However, previous research has found certain socioeconomic factors to be most consistently associated with fertility decline, some of which have been singled out for mention here. These include increases in the urban proportion of a country's population, in per capita income, and in women's educational attainment and employment—especially employment of women of childbearing age, 15 to 44 or 49; declines in infant mortality; and crowded housing conditions. The Appendix table (p. 109) presents available data to illustrate trends in these factors (except housing conditions), and in average desired/ideal family size reported in the countries concerned. It should be noted that estimated *national* averages can be misleading. Rich has offered convincing evidence to demonstrate that fertility has failed to decline in some countries where national rates of economic growth have accelerated remarkably in the last decade, e.g., Mexico, Brazil, and Venezuela, while in others significant fertility declines have occurred at relatively low national levels of per capita income and in rural as well as urban areas. The crucial motivating factor appears to be the extent to which all segments of the population share in the benefits of socioeconomic progress, particularly health services and education (190).

Similarly, Berent points out that in Eastern Europe reported per capita incomes do not adequately indicate relatively high family living standards bolstered by a high proportion of working wives and substantial social welfare benefits—"nonemployment" income (17). Also, detailed research has shown that fertility declines are more closely associated with increasing women's employment where such employment takes women out of the household or the agricultural labor force (134, 189), distinctions that are not usually evident in national estimates of proportions of women in the labor force.

Upward trends in fertility may stem from government pronatalist policies

[b]McIntyre points out that "the introduction of extremely safe, inexpensive and socially sanctioned abortion, offering almost absolute certainty of success at a mortality risk lower than that of actually bearing a child and without the various psycho-sensual drawbacks associated with prior methods of fertility control" may drastically transform the full "costs" of avoidance of births, and thus in itself encourage reductions in desired family size (139, p. 61).

Similarly, the introduction of effective modern contraception (pills, IUDs, and sterilization), whether through private channels or organized family planning programs, may demonstrate to many couples for the first time the possibility of effectively and relatively easily controlling conception and thus in itself contribute to the motivation for fertility control.

(family, maternal and tax benefits and the like) or an increase in sexual activity. Also, average desired family size may fail to decline significantly because of a persistent desire for sons, as in Taiwan and the Republic of Korea.

Demographically, crude birth rates (annual numbers of live births per 1000 population), as used mainly in this report to facilitate international comparisons, can be affected by shifts in a population's age, sex, and rural-urban composition, and in ages at marriage. So far as possible, these factors are also noted where relevant to the situations discussed.

Model for Treatment of Factors Most Relevant to Assessing the Impact of Abortion (Legislation) on Observed Fertility Trends

Table 1-1 sums up the factors mentioned so far that represent some of the most salient that must be considered in attempting to assess the impact of abortion (legalization) on observed fertility trends.

Within this framework, evidence is briefly presented from a number of different countries or areas illustrative of the following situations:

Legal status of abortion changed abruptly from restrictive *to* permissive:

(1) where modern contraception not widely practiced: Eastern Europe, the U.S.S.R., Japan;
(2) where modern contraception widely practiced (or available): New York City, People's Republic of China.

Permissive abortion legally restricted: Romania, Czechoslovakia, Bulgaria.

Legal status of abortion changed (gradually or abruptly) from restrictive *to* moderate, *with increasing reliance on modern contraception: Scandinavia, Great Britain, Singapore, California, Maryland, Washington state.*

Abortion illegal but widely practiced:

(1) where modern contraception increasingly widespread: United States before 1967, Great Britain before 1967, Switzerland, The Netherlands, Republic of Korea, Taiwan;
(2) where modern contraception not yet widely practiced: parts of Western Europe, Israel (Jewish population), Latin America.

It is recognized that these examples represent a variety of different cultures and that extrapolation from the consequences of a legal system in one culture to

Table 1-1

Model for Treatment of Factors Most Relevant to Assessing the Impact of Abortion (Legislation) on Observed Fertility Trends

Independent Variables	Intervening Variables	Dependent Variables
Legal status of abortion: completely restrictive liberalized to varying degrees up to abortion on request	Administrative practices and interpretation of the law De facto availability of abortion services	Changes in observed crude birth rates and/or other fertility rates where feasible
Liberal legislation restricted	Contraceptive practice before and after abortion liberalization	Changes in levels of legal and illegal abortion
	Demographic factors relevant to observed trends in crude birth rate: age/sex/rural-urban structure of population age at marriage	Changes in characteristics of aborters (i.e., young, unmarried, childless versus older, married women with children)
	Family-size preferences relevant to observed fertility trends, influenced by: women's labor force participation and education urbanization per capita income level and growth infant mortality housing conditions government pronatalist policies sex preferences	Changes in levels of out-of-wedlock and premaritally conceived fertility
	Changes in sexual activity	

the likely consequences in quite another culture must be made with caution (33, pp. 218-19). However, there is evidence that whatever the culture, societies and individuals tend to display similar types of abortion-fertility behavior in similar situations.

2 Trends Following Institution of Permissive Abortion

The most rapid recorded declines in fertility have been observed in areas moving abruptly from restrictive to permissive and widely used abortion (33, p. 291; 195, pp. 33-34).

Eastern Europe and the U.S.S.R.

Abortion Liberalization–De Jure and De Facto

The U.S.S.R. pioneered in liberalization of repressive abortion laws when abortion at the request of the pregnant woman was authorized in 1920. Low birth rates prompted a restrictive decree in 1936, but this was repealed in 1955 to combat high levels of illegal abortion–"the harm caused to the health of women by abortions carried out outside hospitals"–and to "give women the possibility of deciding themselves the question of motherhood" (preamble to the Soviet decree, quoted in Field [75, p. 426]). For the same reasons all the Socialist countries of Eastern Europe except the German Democratic Republic and Albania then followed suit: Bulgaria, Hungary, Poland, and Romania in 1956; Czechoslovakia in 1957; and Yugoslavia in 1960 (27, 51, 102, 171, 271). (In the German Democratic Republic, a three-year period of relative permissiveness to deal with increased illegal abortions in the wake of World War II was followed by a strict law in 1950, some permissive interpretation in 1965, and finally legalization of abortion on request in March 1972. According to the first official data released since 1954, the total abortion rate for the following twelve months was 8.4 per 1000 population [58]. This was less than half the comparable Hungarian rate of 19.8 for 1972. However, the GDR birth rate of 11.7 per 1000 population in that year was 15 percent below that of 1971 [13.8], and nearly the world record low for 1972–albeit outdone by the 1972 birth rate of 11.4 in the Federal Republic of Germany, where legal abortion remains restricted.)

From a situation of almost total prohibition (54), abortion became legally available at the request of the woman in the U.S.S.R., Bulgaria, Hungary, and Romania. (In Hungary abortion was already somewhat liberalized in 1953, before becoming available on request in 1956.) A "difficult social situation," backed up only by the word of the pregnant woman herself (since 1960), is acceptable in Poland. In Yugoslavia abortion was authorized "if the birth of the child would result in a serious personal, familial or economic situation for the pregnant woman which cannot be averted in any other way." While abortion requests must be submitted to a board of two physicians (including a gynecologist) and a social worker, only some 10 percent are refused (116). Czechoslovakia required that the woman present specific indications but the criteria were not difficult to meet, except from the end of 1962 to early 1966, when official alarm at low birth and high abortion rates led to temporarily stricter legal interpretation, particularly for women with fewer than three children (33, p. 232; 54, p. 165). (Stricter legal interpretation was again officially ordered in May 1973 [53].)

Abortion was generally prohibited after three months' pregnancy, except for medical reasons, and if the applicant had undergone an induced abortion during the preceding six months (226), although in Poland, for example, the latter rule "seems easy to avoid" (175). Medical abortions are free, while those done on request or for "social" reasons (over 90 percent of all abortions [175]) require a small fee, except in Poland (225). In Czechoslovakia and Hungary abortions must be performed in hospitals, followed by at least an overnight stay, whereas in Poland and parts of Yugoslavia legal abortions are often performed on an outpatient basis, as was the case in Romania before the 1966 restriction discussed in Chapter 3 (54, 226).

Ensuing Levels of Legal Abortion

Following these law changes (and even before in Hungary and Czechoslovakia, in anticipation of the changes), the incidence of legal abortion in Eastern Europe and the U.S.S.R. rose spectacularly. Figures 2-1 through 2-5 depict the trends in rates of registered abortions (legal plus "others": illegal or spontaneous abortions which lead to hospitalization),[a] in birth rates, and in rates of total registered abortions plus live births (indicative of total pregnancies)[b] for those countries in which official data have been consistently available. Of the countries illustrated, *Hungary's* abortion rate has reached the highest level, peaking at 23.2 per 1000 population in 1969, when it exceeded the birth rate by more than 8

[a]Rates of registered "other" abortions declined or stabilized over the period shown in these five countries, except for a rise in 1963 and 1964 in Czechoslovakia during the period of temporarily tightened administrative procedures for legal abortion, discussed in Chapter 3. Therefore, the line depicting rates of legal plus "other" abortions can be taken as generally indicative of the trend in total abortions following legalization.

[b]Total registered abortions plus live births is a substitute for total pregnancies occurring in a population, ignoring stillbirths, and spontaneous and illegal abortions which do not lead to hospitalization, and, hence, registration. Over time following legalization, numbers of illegal abortions declined and therefore rates based on these figures became more nearly indicative of trends in total pregnancies, assuming constant proportions of pregnancies ending in spontaneous abortions or stillbirths.

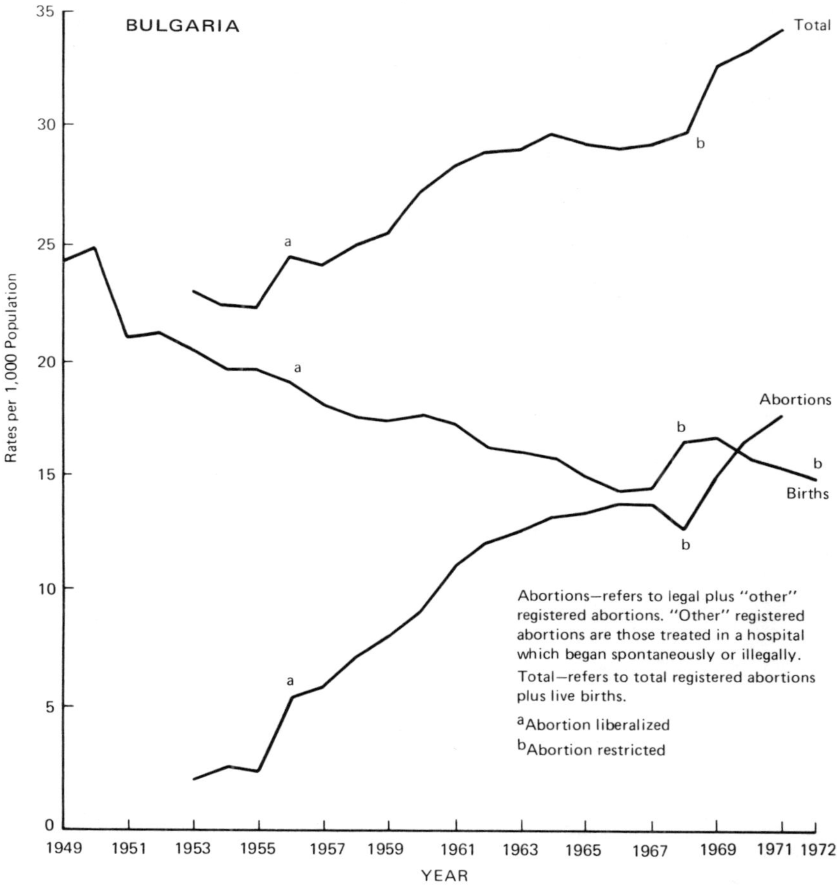

Figure 2-1. Rates per 1,000 Population of Legal and "Other" Registered Abortions, Total Registered Abortions plus Live Births, and Live Births, Bulgaria, 1949-1972. Source: Based on and expanded from figures appearing originally in Myers, p. 93. *Birth rates 1949-52:* H.P. David. *Family planning and abortion in the socialist countries of Central and Eastern Europe.* New York: The Population Council, 1970, table 2, p. 21. *Abortion and birth rates, 1953-72:* H.P. David, M.G. Kalis, and C. Tietze. *Selected abortion statistics: an international summary.* Washington: AIR/Transnational Family Research Institute, 1973 (updated to March 1974). *Total (abortion plus birth) rates:* P.F. Myers. Demographic trends in Eastern Europe. In United States Congress, Joint Economic Committee, *Economic development in countries of Eastern Europe: A compendium of papers.* Washington: U.S. Government Printing Office, 1970, table 10, p. 94 (updated 1967-72 from H.P. David, et al., ibid.).

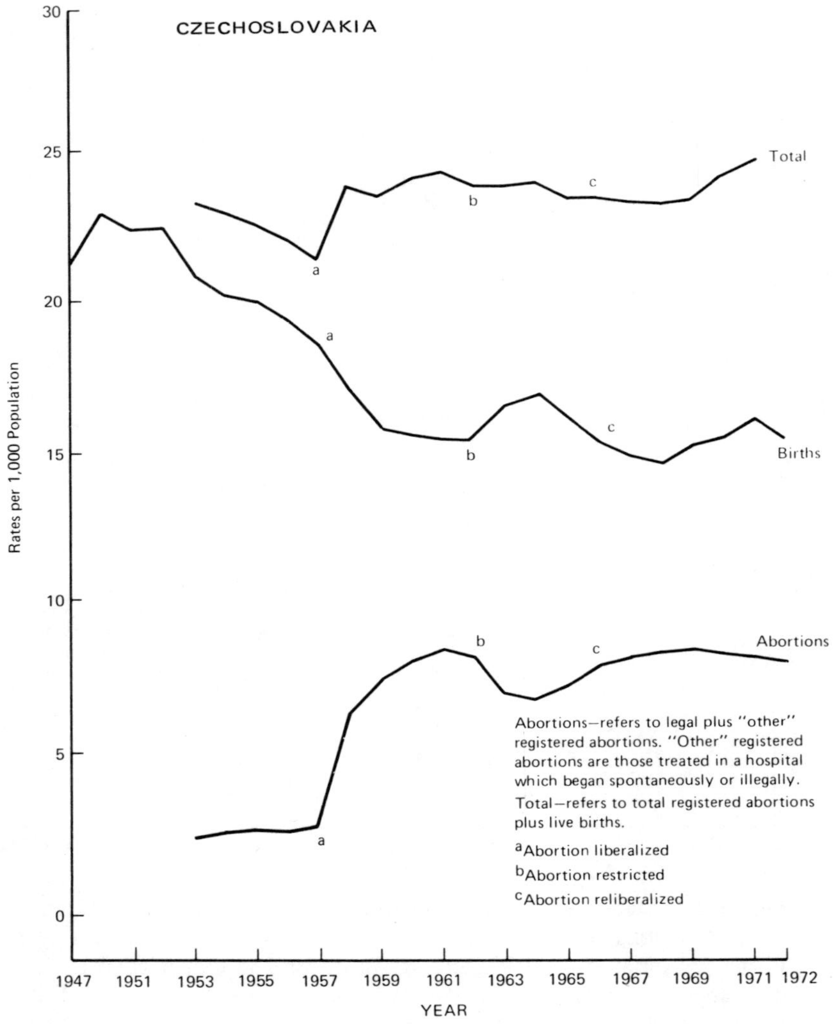

Figure 2-2. Rates per 1,000 Population of Legal and "Other" Registered Abortions, Total Registered Abortions plus Live Births, and Live Births, Czechoslovakia, 1949-1972. Source: Same as Figure 2-1.

points, with a 15 percent decline thereafter to 19.8 in 1972. *Bulgaria's* abortion rate surpassed its crude birth rate for the first time in 1970, and in 1971 stood 2 points higher—18 compared to 16 per 1000 population. Lower abortion rates have been registered in *Yugoslavia, Czechoslovakia*, and *Poland*, in that order. (Abortion data in Poland are probably deficient, due to underregistration of abortions performed by doctors in private practice [175].)

For *Romania*, Mehlan estimated 112,000 and 219,000 legal abortions for the

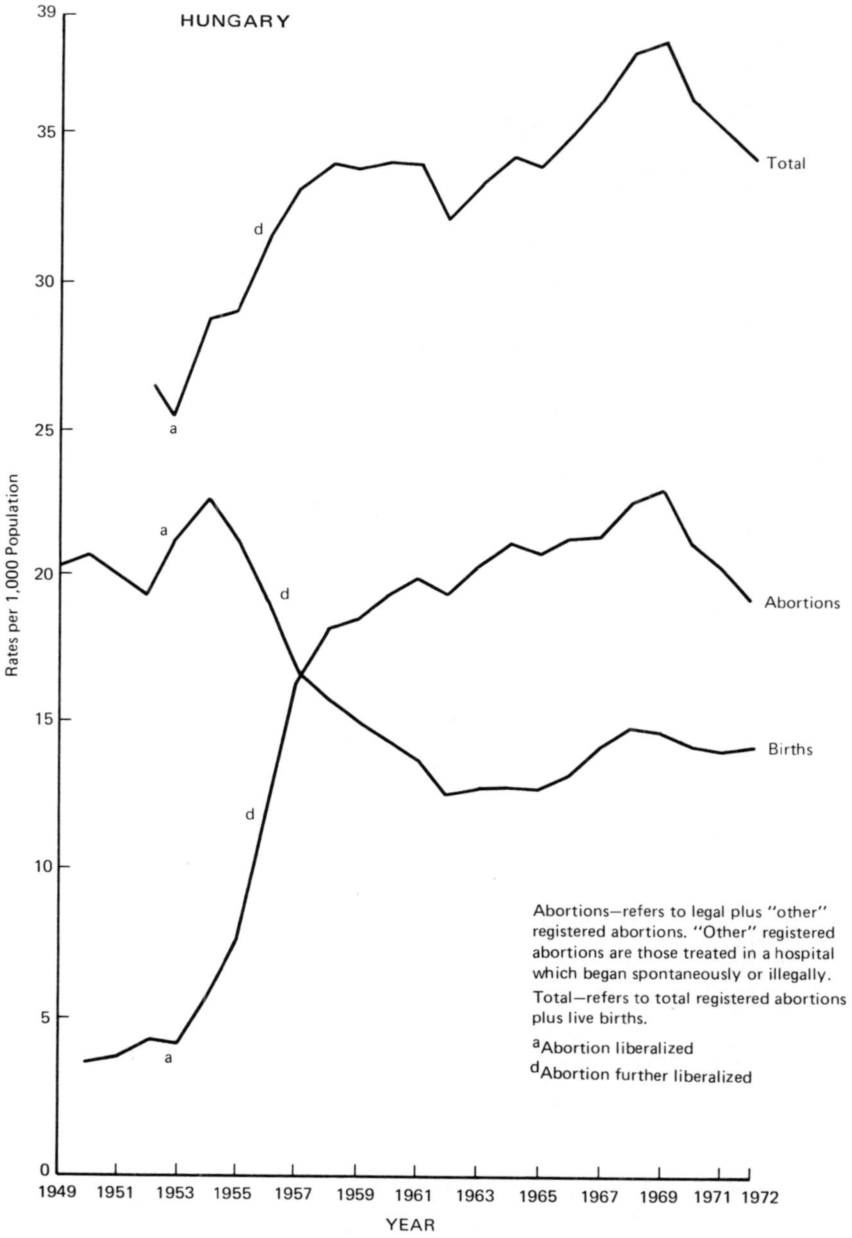

Figure 2-3. Rates per 1,000 Population of Legal and "Other" Registered Abortions, Total Registered Abortions plus Live Births, and Live Births, Hungary, 1949-1972. Source: Same as Figure 2-1.

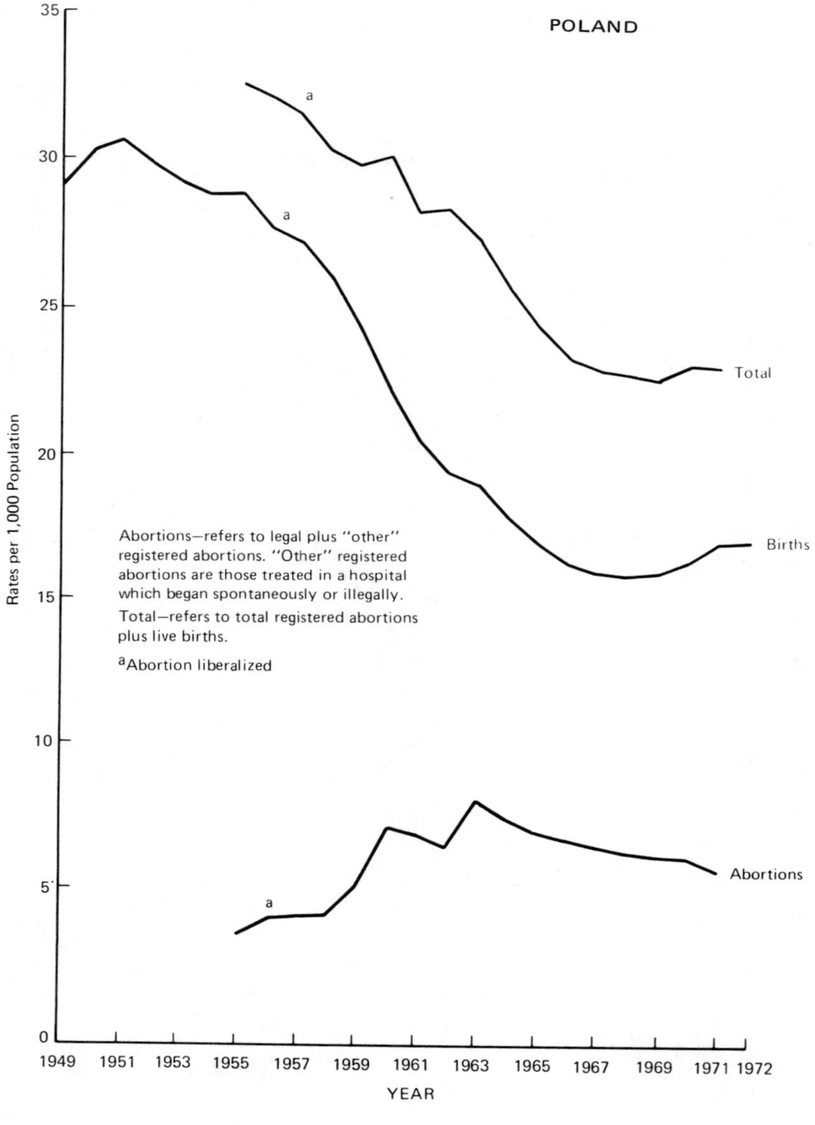

Figure 2-4. Rates per 1,000 Population of Legal and "Other" Registered Abortions, Total Registered Abortions plus Live Births, and Live Births, Poland, 1949-1972. Source: Same as Figure 2-1.

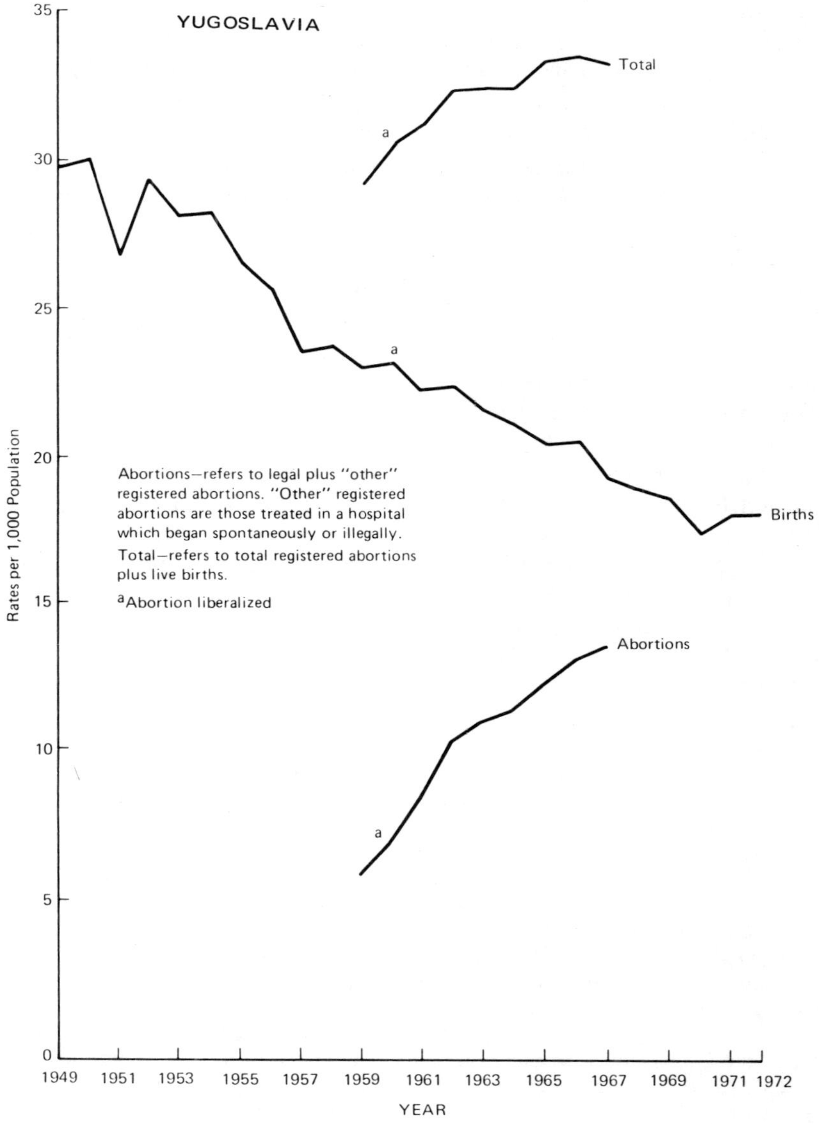

Figure 2-5. Rates per 1,000 Population of Legal and "Other" Registered Abortions, Total Registered Abortions plus Live Births, and Live Births, Yugoslavia, 1949-1972. Source: Same as Figure 2-1.

two years following the 1957 legalization (141). For 1965, the Romanian Communist Party reported 1,115,000 abortions (192)–a total of four abortions for each live birth, the highest incidence of abortion ever reported (152).

In the *U.S.S.R.* abortion data are reportedly collected, but none have been officially published for more than three decades (54, 231). From various sources, Tietze and Dawson estimate that, nationally, abortions (possibly including "hospitalized incomplete") totaled 8.5 million in 1960, 10.6 to 12.8 million in 1965, and over 13 million in 1967, when abortions perhaps outstripped births by more than 3 to 1, for an abortion rate of 56 per 1000 population (231, Table 1)–two and a half times the 1969 Hungarian peak.

Ensuing Birth Rate Trends in Eastern as Compared to Western Europe

A comparison of birth-rate trends in Eastern Europe in the first years following abortion legalization with those in Western Europe, Albania, and the German Democratic Republic, where abortion remained illegal, suggests an abortion effect. Figures 2-6 through 2-8 illustrate trends in crude birth rates, based on the average for the 1950-54 period, in Eastern Europe and seven selected Western and Southern European countries: Belgium, France, Greece, Italy, The Netherlands, Switzerland, and the United Kingdom.

In 1964, Tietze observed:

> By the early 1960s, the birth rate had declined markedly in each of the countries where abortion had been legalized, except in the U.S.S.R. Compared with the early 1950s, the decline ranged from one-fifth in Bulgaria to almost two-fifths in Hungary [Figures 2-6 and 2-7]. Over the same period a moderate increase of natality occurred in several . . . Western countries [e.g., Belgium, Italy, Switzerland, and the United Kingdom, Figure 2-8], as well as in the two Eastern countries which had not legalized abortion [Albania and the German Democratic Republic, Figure 2-7]. Other countries in Western Europe experienced a decline in the birth rate but none by more than one-tenth [Figure 2-8]. The differences in natality trends between the two groups of countries have been sufficiently striking, in my opinion, and the basic patterns of population structure, including its distribution by sex and age, as well as relative changes in per capita income and other indicators of social well-being over the past several years, sufficiently similar, to justify the conclusion, without more rigorous analysis, that the legalization of abortion has had a depressant effect on the birth rate in most of the countries concerned. (225, p. 124)

Table 2-1 displays some data available to illustrate "changes in per capita income" and "other indicators of social well-being" during this period (about 1955-65) in Eastern Europe and the seven Western European countries included in Figure 2-8. Nortman has warned that no perfect yardstick exists by which to measure economic development or to draw quantitative inferences concerning

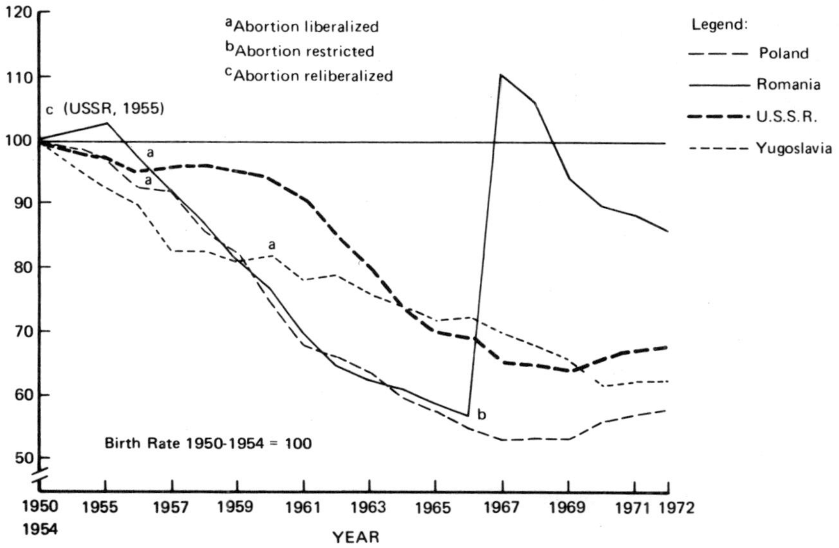

Figure 2-6. Birth Trends in Eastern European Countries, 1950-54 to 1972. Source: Patterned after similar figures in A.R. Omran. Abortion in the demographic transition. In R. Revelle (ed.), *Rapid population growth: Consequences and policy implications.* Vol. 2. Baltimore: The Johns Hopkins Press, 1971, figure 7, p. 523. Derived from basic data given in United Nations, Statistical Office. *Demographic yearbooks.* New York: Author, various years; United Nations, Statistical Office. *Population and vital statistics report: Data available as of 1 October 1973.* New York: Author, Statistical Papers, Series A, Vol. 25, Nos. 3 and 4, 1973; Population Reference Bureau. *1972 World population data sheet.* Washington: Author, 1972.

social and economic well-being (156: 1969, p. 2). In addition, there are well-known drawbacks to attempting international comparisons in all the indicators included in this table (beyond the fact that data are not always available for the same year): women as percent of total labor force, school enrollment, percent urban of total population, per capita income increases, and levels of infant mortality. Given these caveats, it is nevertheless noticeable that a wide range exists in socioeconomic indicators among the countries under consideration. For instance, in the 1960-65 period, the proportion of women in the total labor force ranged from a high of 49 in the U.S.S.R. (1964) to a low of 22 in The Netherlands (1960), although by the end of the 1960s the Eastern European countries (including the German Democratic Republic, where abortion had been somewhat liberalized by this time) did appear to have higher

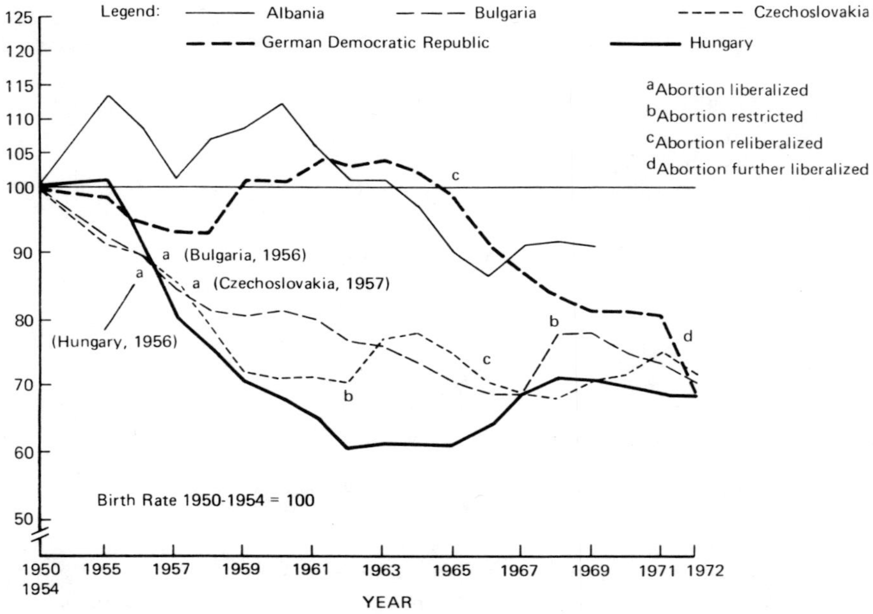

Figure 2-7. Birth Trends in Eastern European Countries, 1950-54 to 1972. Source: Same as Figure 2-6.

proportions of working women than those of the West. School enrollment (indicated by the school enrollment ratio) increased by 89 percent in Romania, 44 percent in Yugoslavia and 36 percent in England and Wales between 1950 and 1965, but by only 7 percent in Hungary and The Netherlands (where it was already a high 85 percent in 1950), and appeared to *decline* in the U.S.S.R. according to the data presented here. Infant mortality rates were generally higher and urbanized proportions of the population generally lower in the East than in the West (and the German Democratic Republic)–two factors which would tend to be associated with *higher* fertility levels, although this does not take account of *changes* in these indicators, which as Berent has observed (below) occurred particularly rapidly in Eastern Europe following World War II. Between 1960 and 1966-67, economic growth (measured by the annual percentage increase in Gross National Product or Gross Domestic Product) appeared to be particularly rapid in low-income countries–Bulgaria and Romania in the East, and Greece among the "Western" group–but other countries displayed similar growth rates. Actual per capita income levels were probably lower in Eastern than in Western Europe in this period (as generally in 1970), but this fails to take account of nonearned income–social welfare

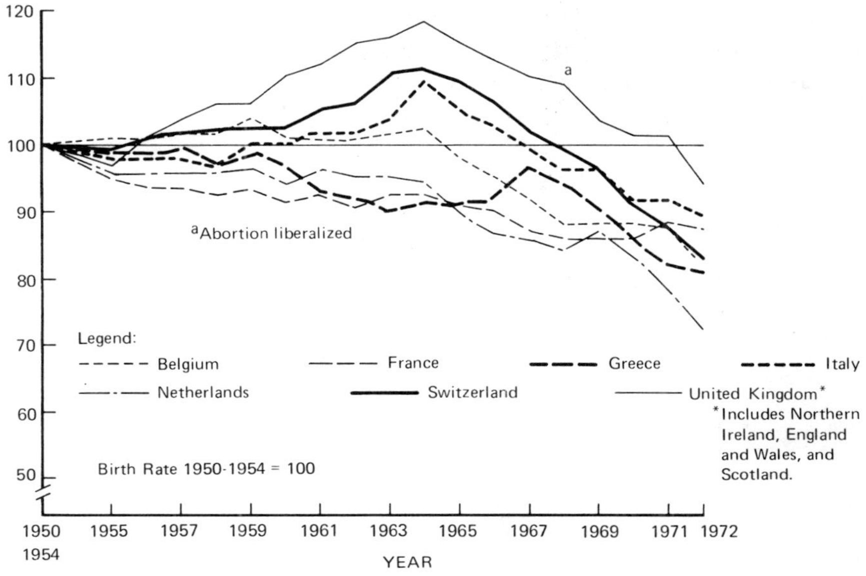

Figure 2-8. Birth Trends in Seven Western European Countries, 1950-54 to 1972. Source: Same as Figure 2-6.

benefits which, as noted, bolstered living standards. Also, urban housing shortages were probably more severe in Eastern than in Western Europe during this period of rapid rural-urban migration in the East (17).

For Eastern Europe, in fact, Myers has observed that the degree of convergence of Eastern Europe's birth rates at a low level by about 1967 was "surprising in view of the *differences* [italics added] that still exist between the countries with respect to those factors that presumably are related to fertility behavior," including levels of living and education, urbanization, industrialization, housing shortages and the extent to which women are employed outside the home (152, p. 90). He regards the underlying reason for this convergence as "the incorporation of the small-family ideal among a large proportion of the population," and remarks that "the relaxation of laws governing abortions was the crucial government action enabling the population of Eastern Europe to attain its desired number of children" (152, pp. 90, 91).

It should be noted that, although birth rates declined faster in the East where abortion had been legalized than in those countries where it had not, birth rates were already declining in Eastern Europe (including Romania and the U.S.S.R.) in the years immediately preceding the law changes, although with some annual fluctuations (Figures 2-1 through 2-5). The annual rate of decline appears to have accelerated initially in Czechoslovakia, Hungary, Poland, and Romania, but

Table 2-1
Selected Socioeconomic Indicators in Eastern Europe and Seven Selected Western European Countries, about 1950-70

		Eastern Europe					
Indicator	Year	Albania	Bulgaria	Czechoslovakia	German Democratic Republic	Hungary	Poland
Women as percent of total labor force					33 (1950)	24 (1950)	31 (1950)
Percent (year)		42 (1955)		35 (1953)			
		39 (1960)	32 (1959)				
				45 (1964)	47 (1964)	38 (1965)	36 (1964)
			43 (1970)	46 (1970)	49 (1970)	43 (1970)	40 (1970)
Adjusted school enrollment ratio[b]	1950	68	63	76	84	77	70
Both sexes	1965	90	88	80	103	82	88
Percent urban of total population			28 (1950)	52 (1950)	71 (1950)	38 (1950)	37 (1950)
Percent (year)		32 (1962)	38 (1960)	57 (1960)	72 (1960)	42 (1960)	48 (1960)
Gross national product (GNP)[c] per capita in US $	1960						
	1970	600	760	2,230	2,490	1,600	1,400
GNP per capita, annual percent increase	1955-60		6.3	5.4	5.8	3.5	2.9
	1960-67		6.0	2.4	3.0	4.2	3.6
	1960-70	4.8	7.4	3.8	4.2	5.4	5.2
Real gross domestic product (GDP)[c] per capita, annual percent increase	1960-66						
Infant deaths per 1000 live births		81.5 (1964)	32.9 (1964)	25.5 (1965)	28.8 (1964)	40.0 (1964)	54.8 (1960)
Rate (year)			27.3 (1970)	22.9 (1969)	19.0 (1970)	35.7 (1970)	33.4 (1970)

			Western Europe						
Romania	U.S.S.R.	Yugoslavia	Belgium	France	Greece	Italy	Netherlands	Switzerland	United Kingdom
					18 (1951)	26 (1951)		30 (1950)	31[a] (1951)
		25 (1956)		34 (1954)			21 (1956)		
27 (1960)			27 (1961)	35 (1962)	33 (1961)	25 (1961)	22 (1960)	30 (1960)	
	49 (1964)							29 (1965)	38[a] (1966)
30 (1970)		30 (1968)	31 (1968)	35 (1968)		27 (1968)			
47	83	55	84	78	70	53	85	64	75[a]
89	82	79	93	91	81	70	91	64	102[a]
25 (1950)									
32 (1960)	51 (1962)	28 (1961)		63 (1962)	44 (1961)	48 (1961)	76 (1962)	51 (1960)	80[a] (1962)
	1,160			1,960		1,100	1,675		1,855
930	1,790	650	2,720	3,100	1,090	1,760	2,430	3,320	2,270
3.1		6.2							
5.7		3.9							
7.7	5.8	4.3	4.0	4.6	6.6	4.6	3.9	2.5	2.2
			3.9	3.9	6.7	4.7			2.2
52.0 (1964)	29.4 (1964)	75.8 (1964)	25.3 (1964)	23.3 (1964)	35.8 (1964)	36.1 (1964)	14.8 (1964)	21.1 (1960)	22.5 (1960)
49.5 (1970)	24.4 (1970)	49.0 (1971)	21.7 (1970)	20.1 (1966-70)	31.8 (1969)	29.2 (1970)	12.4 (1970)	16.1 (1969)	18.8 (1968)

Table 2-1 (notes)

Sources:

Women as percent of total labor force: J. Berent, *Some demographic aspects of female employment in Eastern Europe.* London: International Union for the Scientific Study of Population, 1969, table 1, p. B4; E. Szabady, Interdependence between changes in fertility and the socio-economic development of Eastern European countries. Unpublished paper. Budapest: Demographic Institute of the Hungarian Central Statistical Office, 1972, table 3, p. 7; United Nations. *Demographic yearbook 1970.* New York: United Nations Statistical Office, 1971, table 12, p. 595.

Adjusted school enrollment ratio: United Nations Economic and Social Council (UNESCO). *Statistical yearbook 1967.* Paris: Author, 1968, table 2.5, p. 72.

Percent urban of total population: Szabady, op.cit., table 2, p. 6; United Nations, op.cit., table 5, p. 136.

Gross National Product: World Bank. *World Bank atlas: Population, per capita product and growth rates.* Washington: Author, 1972; World Bank. *Trends in developing countries.* Washington: Author, 1973, tables 2.5 and 2.7.

GNP annual percent increase: T.P. Alton, Economic structure and growth in Eastern Europe. In United States Congress, Joint Economic Committee, *Economic developments in countries of Eastern Europe: A compendium of papers.* Washington: U.S. Government Printing Office, 1970, table 3, p. 47; World Bank atlas, op.cit.

Real gross domestic product per capita, annual percent increase; United Nations. *Statistical yearbook 1967.* New York, Author, 1968.

Infant deaths per 1000 live births: United Nations. *Demographic yearbook 1968.* New York: United Nations Statistical Office, 1969, table 17, p. 366; International Planned Parenthood Federation. *Situation Reports.* London: Author, various countries, most recent issues.

[a]England and Wales.

[b]This ratio is based on the total enrollment in the first and second levels of education related to the estimated population 5-19 years old; it is adjusted to correspond to the actual duration of schooling. The ratio may be regarded as a rough indicator of the enrollment status of a given country, but should be used cautiously in international comparisons. For a fuller description, see the original source, UNESCO, *Statistical yearbook*, 1967. Paris, 1968, p. 7. Nortman, D. Population and family planning programs: A factbook. *Reports on Population/Family Planning*, December 1969, p. 29, note 10.

[c]*Gross domestic product* (GDP) represents the contribution of each resident producer in a country to the total production of the country. At market prices, it is the market value of the product. However, not all producers are residents of the country, and some residents produce outside the country. When gross domestic product is adjusted for these inward and outward flows of factor income, the result is known as *gross national product* (GNP). For further detail, see definition of terms in any annual issue of United Nations, *Yearbook of national accounts statistics.* Nortman, ibid., September 1972, p. 29, note 23.

was more gradual in Yugoslavia, and delayed in the U.S.S.R. (below). (In Hungary, as revealed in Figure 2-3, the birth rate had risen markedly in 1952 and 1953 during a concerted campaign against illegal abortion [138].) However, the drop of 21 percent in Bulgaria's birth rate in the nine years from 1955—the last full year before the 1956 abortion law change—to 1964 (20.0 to 16.1 per 1000 population), was less than the 25 percent noted by Sweezy for the nine years from 1920-21 to 1929 (40.0 to 30.1 per 1000 population [220]). Also, Yugoslavia's birth rate had dropped 13 percent in the five years from 1952 to 1956 (29.7 to 25.9), compared to an 8 percent drop that occurred in the five years dating from just before the 1960 law change in that country—1959 to 1963 (23.3 to 21.4 per 1000).

In the *U.S.S.R. and Yugoslavia*, reported national statistical averages mask the impact of induced abortion on fertility. In both countries there are vast regional differences in birth and abortion rates (59), with low fertility generally associated with high abortion levels and vice versa. For example, in a 1970 fertility survey of married Yugoslavian women, the percentage admitting to ever having had an abortion was 66 in Vojvodina and 62 in Serbia (relatively more prosperous areas), compared to only 21 in less-developed Kosova. General fertility rates (births per 1000 women aged 15 to 44) in the year preceding the survey were 50 in Vojvodina, 55 in Serbia, and 174 in Kosovo (25).

McIntyre has reckoned that removing the *effects of structural changes* that would tend to depress crude birth rates (shifts in age, sex, and rural-urban composition of the population, and nuptiality patterns) leaves a "pure" fertility drop of 31 percent in Bulgaria and 83 percent in Hungary between 1955 and 1965, and 54 percent in Czechoslovakia between 1955 and 1962 (138, Table 9-7).

A partial exception to the pattern of more rapid birth rate declines in the East than in the West in this period is the *U.S.S.R.*, where a marked birth-rate decline became evident only half a decade after the 1955 abortion reliberalization (Figure 2-6). One possibility is that many abortions were done but were offset by a gradual equalization of the sex ratio after World War II. High marriage rates were registered (about 12 per 1000 population between 1956 and 1960), and a continuous decline in the proportion of husbandless women would have compensated for the effects of rising abortion rates. Urban areas, where abortion rates are high have lower birth rates than rural areas, where abortion rates are lower, which supports the findings (17; 195, p. 34). Heer also suggests that in the late 1950s many legal abortions merely replaced illegal abortions. In general, however, he feels that "legalization of abortion has no doubt been a very important factor in the decline of Soviet fertility" (95, p. 233), although the drop in birth rates following reliberalization in 1955 has never been so steep or sudden as the rise following the 1936 restriction.

Concomitant Contraceptive Use in Eastern Europe and the U.S.S.R.

Coitus interruptus evidently remains the most widely used contraceptive method throughout Eastern Europe and the U.S.S.R., as in the past, despite increasing availability of IUDs and pills as from the late 1960s (and as early as 1964 in Yugoslavia [116]) and increasing promotion of family planning (designed to combat high rates of abortion) in some countries. Surveys also reveal that a high percentage of aborters have relied on coitus interruptus, e.g., 69 percent in a

1966 Bulgarian study (54). Peel and Potts attribute the long-time condemnation of coitus interruptus as the most unreliable of contraceptive methods to the "esthetic biases . . . [of] middleclass commentators." They point out that this method played an important part in the demographic transition of Europe in the eighteenth and nineteenth centuries, and that British, American, and Indian studies reveal that its failure rate can be equal to or less than that of diaphragms and condoms, and very much less than that of rhythm (168, pp. 49-50). However, on the basis of twelve-month failure rates recorded in the 1965 National Fertility Study in the United States, Jaffe rates coitus interruptus as a "least effective" method in actual use, along with rhythm, foam, jelly, douching, and suppositories. Diaphragms and condoms are rated as "moderately effective," while the pill and IUD are "most effective" (110, Table 2).

In *Hungary*, 63 percent of married women reported current use of any contraceptive method in a 1966 nationwide survey. Among these, 62 percent relied on coitus interruptus. Rhythm, douching, or abstinence were used by another 9 percent. It was estimated that 58 percent of all the women surveyed had had at least one induced abortion, although only 13 percent relied on abortion alone to control fertility. Two-fifths of the women had never received any information on contraception (2). (In 1974, along with partial repeal of elective abortion, contraceptive instruction before marriage will become mandatory in Hungary, and will be officially provided together with sex education for school children of all ages, their parents, and the general population [103].) That a shift to modern contraception may now be occurring in Hungary is evident from national estimates of rising numbers of women using pills, which were introduced in 1967 (e.g., a 66 percent increase from 133,000 to 170,000 between December 1969 and December 1970 [108]), and from data collected in a longitudinal study of 5 percent of all women married in 1966. By 1972, 36 percent of these women (first interviewed on the day of their marriage in 1966 and twice since then) reported current use of the pill. This may be more attributable to increasing age, duration of marriage, and numbers of children than wider availability of modern contraception. Some 42 percent were still using "traditional methods"—coitus interruptus, abstinence, and rhythm (123). However, the downturn in the abortion rate since 1969 *and* in the birth rate (to at least 1971)[c] and pregnancy rate (total of registered abortions plus births) suggests that modern contraception is indeed now replacing abortion as the principal means of fertility control in Hungary (Figure 2-3). The availability of easy abortion may have retarded this development, as indicated by the fact that 78 percent of Budapest women recently interviewed in abortion surveys replied that they would resort to more effective contraceptive methods than currently used if the prevailing permissive abortion system were to be abolished (221).

[c]Despite the 1967 extension and subsequent heavy use of paid maternity leaves for working women to three years after childbirth, in addition to many other pronatalist incentives (17, 140).

Among married women sampled nationwide in *Czechoslovakia*, "preference for" coitus interruptus was expressed by 75 percent in 1956 and declined to 43 percent in 1959, but in 1970 this method was still used by 33 percent among lower classes and 42 percent among upper classes (54, p. 174; 210, Table 25). By 1970, IUDs were employed by 23 percent of upper-class married women and 14 percent in the lower classes, with pill use reported by only 8 percent in the upper classes and 5 percent in lower classes. The resort to abortion had evidently stabilized. The proportion of women admitting to having had at least one abortion was the same in 1970 as in 1959–20 percent.

In *Yugoslavia*, results of the first countrywide family-planning survey conducted in 1970 indicated that 45 percent of married women had had an induced abortion (25) and thus, "abortion is the most frequently used method of limiting family size in Yugoslavia" (116, p. 183). Some 44 percent used no contraception, 38 percent used coitus interruptus, 3.6 percent the pill, and 1 percent the IUD. The low pill use is surprising in view of the fact that in this period in Croatia, for example, the total cost of an abortion was estimated to be equivalent to that of a five-year pill supply (212). Residual medical opposition to modern contraceptive methods is suggested as a possible cause for the apparently slow shift to IUDs and pills in Yugoslavia (180).

Official family-planning programs have been more vigorous over a longer period in *Poland* than in the rest of Eastern Europe (54). The first family-planning clinic opened in 1928; the International Planned Parenthood Federation-affiliated Polish Family Planning Association currently has branches throughout the country, and there are more than 3000 family-planning consultation centers. Every new mother is required to receive family-planning instruction, and the social security system covers 70 percent of the cost of contraceptives. The success of these programs is evident in the rapidly falling trend of pregnancies (abortions plus live births) seen in Figure 2-4, associated with the lowest abortion rates of the countries. This figure and Figure 2-2 for Czechoslovakia show *upward* trends in birth rates to at least 1971 (and leveling or downturns in abortion rates) for these two countries since 1967-68, possibly in response to the increased intensity of government pronatalist policies–extensions of maternal leave, family allowances, and maternity grants since 1968 in Czechoslovakia in particular (17).

Romania's extreme level of abortion in 1965 suggests that this was virtually the sole method of fertility regulation before the October 1966 restriction (see Chapter 3). However, Moore-Cavar points out that even the 1,115,000 abortions reported for 1965 amounted to only 59 per 1000 of the country's then population–far less than the rate of 72 to 108 per 1000 that would have been required in a noncontracepting population (2 to 3 abortions per live birth–see Introduction) to reduce unrestricted natural fertility rates of about 50 births per 1000 population to the 14.3 observed in Romania in September 1966. Therefore, she surmises that coitus interruptus, abstinence, and prolonged breast-feeding were widely practiced in addition to abortion (146, Chapter 11).

In the *U.S.S.R.*, despite public and medical opposition to the widespread use of abortion as a health hazard, fragmentary evidence suggests that modern contraceptives are not widely available; that locally manufactured condoms, though cheap, are of poor quality and hence disliked; and that coitus interruptus remains the most frequent method of contraception, if any (56).

Socioeconomic Development, Housing Conditions, and Desired Family Size

Berent has well reviewed the impact on fertility of the post-World War II increases in industrialization, urbanization, real family income, and levels of education and women's employment, as well as declines in infant mortality, that occurred in Eastern Europe (17; see also Appendix table). He feels that the unrivaled *speed* of these changes, coupled with severe housing shortages (continued doubling-up of families and a rigorous policy of building only small apartments) largely explains why surveys of the 1960s indicate that the overwhelming majority of couples considered one or two children ideal. So long as contraceptive practices remained poorly developed it is to be expected that easily available, socially sanctioned abortion contributed considerably to the close fit achieved in this region between actual and desired family size.

Japan

Abortion Liberalization–De Jure and De Facto

From a situation of strict prohibition of abortion, comparable to that in Eastern Europe before liberalization, Japan moved to "beyond doubt, the most permissive abortion system in the world" (33, p. 253) by 1952, when two amendments to the 1948 Eugenic Protection Law authorized abortions for economic as well as health reasons and left the decision regarding abortions "entirely at the discretion" of those physicians specially designated to perform them. In 1967 it was reported that these physicians numbered some 13,000 and "are usually within easy reach in any locality" (148). The cost was then no more than U.S. $15 for first-trimester abortions (147)–all but 5 percent of reported abortions in recent years (231, Table 16)–using dilatation and curettage, which is still the preferred method for early abortions in Japan (231). For the 70 percent of the Japanese population covered by public health insurance, induced abortions permitted for health reasons could be reduced to less than $1 (147).

As in Eastern Europe, the officially expressed aim of liberalization was to safeguard women's health in view of rapidly rising numbers of criminal abortions, as well as "to prevent the increase of inferior descendants from the standpoint of eugenic protection" (113). Concern with population trends, even in the prevailing seriously overcrowded postwar situation, was not an officially declared objective, although "liberalized abortion was expected to accelerate the desired process of fertility decline (149, p. 6).

Ensuing Levels of Legal Abortion

According to official reports, numbers of abortions in Japan following legalization rose from 246,000 in 1949 to a peak of 1.17 million in 1955 (112), representing a legal abortion rate of 13.1 compared to a birth rate of 19.4 per 1000 population in that year. Underreporting of abortions is recognized as widespread, which has been attributed partially to private physicians apparently wishing to avoid income taxes (257). Independent investigations estimate the true incidence of abortions as from 1.5 to 3.7 times the reported numbers (150), on the basis of which Tietze and Dawson estimate that the ratio of abortions to 1000 live births six months later ranged between 1800 and 2200 between 1955 and 1965 (231, Table 1). However, from about 1960 there probably has been a real decline in abortions,[d] together with increasingly widespread and effective contraception (see below) *and*—since 1961— slightly rising birth rates (Figure 2-9). The one exception is perhaps 1966, the "Year of the Fiery Horse." According to tradition, girls born during such a year grow up to be bad-natured and hence difficult to marry off. In that year the birth rate dropped precipitously (Figure 2-9). Tietze and Lewit suggest that "since it is doubtful that the sharp drop in births can be attributed mainly to a surge in the effective use of contraception by the most traditionbound segment of Japanese society, one can surmise that the number of abortions must actually have risen, rather than declined, in 1966" (232, p. 26). Aso argues, however, that rather than an increase in (unreported) abortions, the 1966 birth dip was indeed due to a marked increase in contraception and some misreporting of birth dates for girl babies (12). A series of eleven nationwide fertility surveys by the Population Problems Research Council of the Mainichi Newspapers shows a peak of 56 percent of women reporting current contraceptive use in 1965, which fell off to 53 percent in 1967 (172: 1971, Table III-1). Also, as in 1906, the previous Fiery Horse Year, the sex ratio of officially reported births rose to a suspiciously high level—107.6 male per 100 female babies, compared to a long-constant sex ratio ranging between 104 and 105—suggesting that many parents anxious to avoid the Fiery Horse Year curse "adjusted" dates reporting actual 1966 female births.

[d]However, after declining to 732,000 in 1970, *reported* abortions rose to 739,000 in 1971 (231, Table 1).

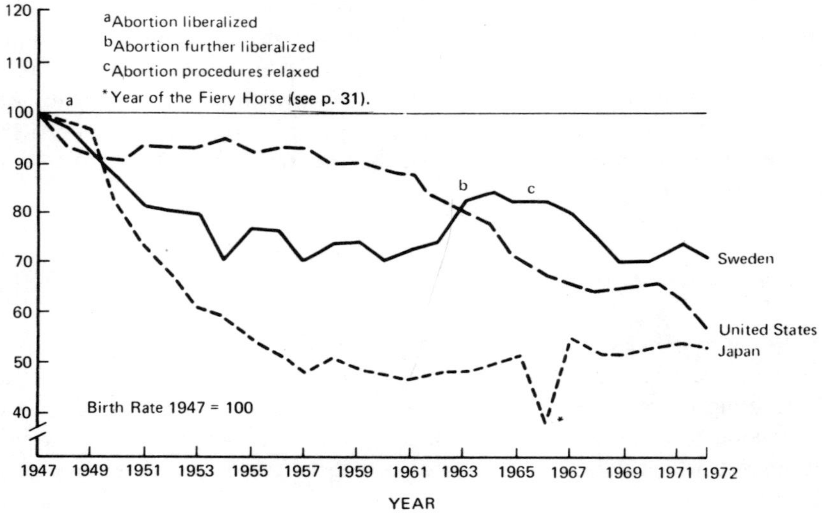

Figure 2-9. Birth Trends in Japan, Sweden, and the United States, 1947-72. Source: Same as Figure 2-6.

In the series of Mainichi Newspapers national surveys, the percentage of currently married women under 50 admitting to having had at least one abortion rose from 15 in 1952 to 41 in 1961, and dropped thereafter to 37 in 1971. (Tietze and Dawson estimate 49 percent for 1971, correcting for underreporting [231, Table 2], but there has probably been a real decline since the 1961 peak in the percentage of women who have had at least one abortion.) These surveys also indicate that abortion was relatively more frequent in urban than in rural areas in Japan before 1961 (540 abortions per 1000 live births in urban areas, compared to 330 in rural areas in 1952), but the relationship had reversed by 1965 (440 compared to 530 respectively). By 1971 there were negligible rural-urban differences in abortion use, and also in family sizes. Also the use of abortion has been shifting downward from higher to lower classes (with more use of contraception in higher classes reported in 1969—see below—and negligible class differences in family size), in conformity with the model illustrated in Figure 1-1. Among women with nine or fewer years of formal schooling, the percentage with abortion experience rose from 12 to 32 between 1962 and 1965, while the comparable percentage among women with 13 plus years of schooling dropped from 37 to 32 in these years (76, Table 9).

Ensuing Birth Rate Trends

In 1963, Davis stated that in Japan "the resort to abortion has been the leading [although not the only] cause of probably the fastest drop in the birth rate ever exhibited by an entire nation" (61, p. 345). In the ten years from 1947 (just before abortion legalization) to 1957, Japan's birth rate dropped by 50 percent, from 34 to 17 per 1000 population—a dramatic difference from the concurrent 22-28 percent drop in Sweden, where legal abortion was then moderately available (see Chapter 4), although Sweden's birth rates were already at a relatively low level (14-18 per 1000), and the scarcely varying level in the United States (25-27 per 1000), where legal abortion remained restricted (Figure 2-9). It should be noted that Japan's 1947 birth rate of 34.3 was a postwar high, somewhat above the level of about 30 per 1000 of the 1930s and wartime years of the early 1940s (240).

Taking into account the number of married women of fertile age, their reproductive activities and level of fecundity, and survey estimates of concurrent contraceptive practice, Muramatsu has estimated that without induced abortion about 2.4 million more births would have occurred in Japan in 1955 than the actual 1.73 million recorded (151).

To demonstrate the impact of legal abortion on rates of population growth (in contrast to birth rates), Burnhill has used U.N. demographic data and reliable country sources of abortion data to calculate expected, as compared to observed, rates of natural increase (birth minus death rates) for Japan and Czechoslovakia for the period 1961 to 1965. Assuming that had abortion not been available in each of these countries 85 percent of the reported abortions would have resulted in live births,[e] he reckons that Japan's rate of natural increase would have been 18.6 per 1000 population rather than the 10.3 observed, and Czechoslovakia's 11.7 compared with the observed 6.6. This would have cut the doubling time of the population at that time from 67 to 37 years in Japan and from 105 to 59 years in Czechoslovakia (30).

Concomitant Contraceptive Use

Among the national samples of Japanese married women, the percentage reporting *current* use of contraception increased steadily, from 20 in 1950, to 34

[e]This is probably an overestimate, given the limited practice of effective contraception in these countries in this period. However, recorded (legal) operations declined in Czechoslovakia in this period (see Chapter 3), due to more stringent regulations, which would counterbalance this to some extent.

in 1955, to a peak of 56 in 1965, and dropped slightly thereafter, as noted. In 1971, only 17 percent had never used contraception, and 53 percent reported current use. Adjusting for misreporting, Tietze and Dawson estimate the 1971 percentage of current contraceptive use by fertile-aged women in Japan as 59 (231, p. 50), which is close to the comparable percentage of 65 reported among currently married women in the United States in 1970 (see Chapter 4). In 1969, 72 percent of college-educated women were practicing contraception, compared to 34 percent of those with only primary education. (Note, however, that in that year 87 percent of Japanese girls of appropriate age were enrolled in secondary school. Appendix table.) Continuing medical opposition virtually prohibits use of pills and IUDs for contraception (9). In 1971, of those practicing contraception, 33 percent used rhythm, 4 percent were sterilized, and 73 percent used condoms (172: 1973, Table 2-5-1. Many couples use more than one method.). Long the most popular method in Japan, condoms are of high quality and aggressively marketed (attractive packaging, door-to-door promotion by women to women [136]), so that their "use" effectiveness is probably very high in comparison to other situations. Muramatsu reckons the antifertility impact of abortion versus contraception as 257 to 100 in 1955. By 1965 the ratio was almost equal, and by 1970 the balance had shifted, with abortion yielding to contraception, according to his calculations, in a ratio of 85 to 100 as a means of averting births (151). Note that, except for 1966, birth rates in Japan also increased gradually to 19.3 per 1000 in 1971, after reaching a low of 16.9 in 1961 (Figure 2-9). Cho and Retherford estimate that nearly half of this rise can be attributed to the increased numbers of postwar baby-boomers reaching prime ages of childbearing (43), which among Japanese women is now almost completely concentrated in the 20-29-year-old age group (183).

Socioeconomic Development and Natural Increase in Japan

Davis considers the spectacular post-World War II economic rise of Japan only part of a process starting long before. During the forty-five years from 1913 to 1958 the average growth rate of industrial output in Japan rose by 5.4 percent per year, exceeding the 5 percent annual increase of Germany and the United States from 1880 to 1913, and greatly exceeding the performance of the United Kingdom and France in any sustained period. (From 1960 to 1970, Japan's Gross National Product per capita growth rate averaged 9.6 percent annually, compared to 3.2 percent in the United States. See Appendix table.) Concurrently, in the thirty years from 1920 to 1950, Japanese mortality rates dropped to an extent that had required seventy-six years in Sweden, resulting in a prolonged period of high natural increase (an average 12.8 per 1000 population annually from 1900 to 1950. Natural increase has again risen to this level in

Japan since 1969, due to rising birth rates. The death rate has remained steady at about 6.8 per 1000 population [240: 1971, Table 30].) Davis argues that the widespread use of abortion was not peculiarly Japanese, arising out of ancient Tokugawa traditions, as has sometimes been suggested, but part of a "multiphasic response" (which also included increasing contraception, delayed marriage, and outmigration before World War II)—not to spreading poverty or national "overpopulation" but to the perceived antagonism between such a high rate of natural increase and the individual family's ability to capitalize on the increasing national prosperity (61). Davis feels such a response was probably also typical of Northern and Western European countries at similar stages of economic development and falling mortality, which implies that the role of abortion merely assumed more visibility in Japan because of its timely legalization. However, the evidence suggests that, thanks to its legalization and wide availability, abortion also assumed more importance in Japan than in the West at a similar stage of development, and that in its contribution to the achievement of lower family sizes, abortion legislation can be considered one cornerstone of Japan's postwar "economic miracle" (180).

New York City

Abortion Liberalization—De Jure and De Facto

Culminating a national movement to bring abortion "from the backrooms to the hospitals and clinics" and permit women the freedom to "control their own fertility" (243, pp. 173, 174), on July 1, 1970, New York state declared "an abortional act justifiable" when performed upon a female *with her consent* by a duly licensed physician acting (a) under a reasonable belief that such is necessary to preserve *her* life, or (b) *within twenty-four weeks from the commencement of her pregnancy* (154. Italics in original). In eliminating all specified indications for abortion, this act was more liberal than the abortion reform laws passed from 1967 to 1970 in twelve other American states (203); and in setting no restrictions on residency of patients or location of the operation, went beyond other "repeal" laws passed in Hawaii, Washington, and Alaska. Even the similarly sweeping U.S. Supreme Court decisions of January 22, 1973 permit state regulation of the location of abortion operations after the first twelve weeks of pregnancy (251). As predicted, New York City in particular quickly became an "abortion mecca." But contrary to "dire prophecies," the city's hospitals developed "in an amazingly short time" the necessary services and staff to care for women requesting abortions (162), joined by the twenty-four freestanding clinics operating by the second year (163).

In the first two years, the cost of an abortion performed on an ambulatory basis (permissible in the first trimester when, by the second year, 82 percent of all abortions to New York City residents occurred [229]) ranged between $150 and $200 (169). Free abortions were supplied by some physicians and facilities to indigent women. Medicaid covered the costs of abortions for registered low-income women until a court ruling of February 1972 (since reversed), which was protested by the city's Health Services, which declared that "no New York City resident would be denied an abortion because of inability to pay" (169, p. 29).

Ensuing Levels of Legal Abortion

Of 402,000 legal abortions performed in the two years following the law change, New York City residents underwent an estimated 67,400 in the first year and 75,100 in the second (229). Before liberalization, in 1965-67, all reported therapeutic abortions in the city averaged 321 annually (70). In that period, legal abortion ratios (numbers of abortions per 1000 live births) for white women were more than twice the ratio for nonwhites. In the first year following liberalization, the ratio for nonwhite women of 774 substantially exceeded that of 418 for white women. Tietze remarks that "while this [latter] differential probably reflects differential success in utilization of the most effective contraceptive methods, it also indicates that legal abortion was now accessible to and utilized by all the city's ethnic and economic groups" (229, p. 41)—a reversal of the situation which had roused major criticism during the earlier restrictive period. (Abortion ratios were far lower among Puerto Ricans in both periods, possibly reflecting the high frequency of contraceptive sterilization among Puerto Rican women who have borne all the children they want, as well as the Catholic Hispanic traditional rejection of abortion [229] .) Tietze also observes that legal abortion rates (abortions per 1000 women aged 15 to 44) among New York City's white and nonwhite residents in the two years following legalization were of the same order of magnitude as the rate of numbers plus timing failures that can be assumed to have occurred among the 1966-70 births to such women according to the results of the 1970 National Fertility Study. (In this study, the percentages of 1966-70 births reported as "unplanned"—number plus timing failures—were 61 percent among blacks and 42 percent among white married women of reproductive age [243, p. 164] .) This suggests that freely available, elective abortion would aid all U.S. women to have the children they want when they want them, which could reduce national fertility to replacement level (see below).

Ensuing Birth Trends in New York City

From 1970 to 1972 annual numbers of live births declined by 33,800–23 percent. The drop was sharper than for the rest of the nation–11.6 and 12.4 percent in 1971 and 1972, compared to 4.3 and 8.8 percent for the United States as a whole (163; Figure 2-10). The decline is especially noteworthy since an increase in births had been predicted for the 1970s because of increased numbers of women of childbearing age stemming from the baby boom of the late 1940s (94). Tietze attributes half of the decline to greater utilization of legal abortion by New York City residents following the July 1970 liberalization of the state law (229).

Out-of-wedlock births dropped by 12 percent between 1970 and 1971–31,900 to 28,000–the first reversal in what had been a steady upward trend since 1954, when data on such births in the city were first collected (229). Tietze observes that "more than one-third of the estimated decline of 15,600 births in 1971 attributable to legal abortion is represented by the decline in out-of-wedlock births" (228, p. 583).

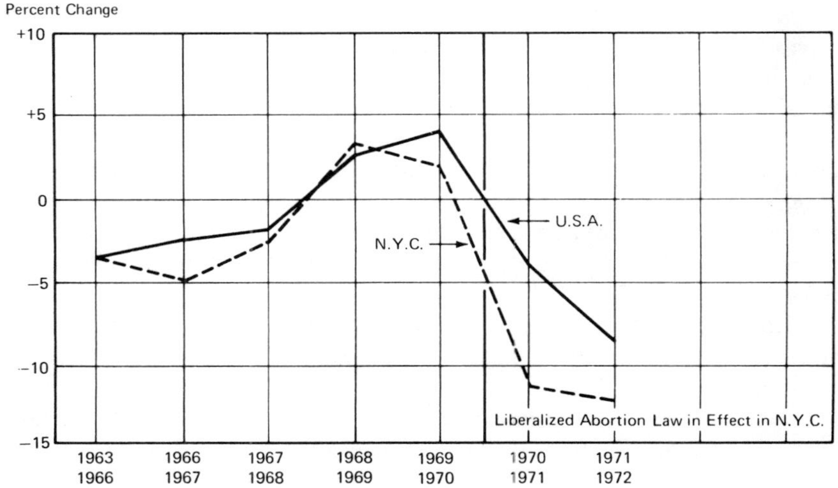

Figure 2-10. Annual Percent Change in Number of Live Births, United States and New York City, 1965 through 1972. Source: J. Pakter, D. O'Hare, F. Nelson, and M. Svigir. Two years' experience in New York City with the liberalized abortion law: progress and problems. *American Journal of Public Health*, 1973, 63, figure 2, p. 533. Reprinted with permission.

Concomitant Contraceptive Use

No separate data on contraceptive practice are available for New York City, but the 1970 National Fertility Study indicated that some 65 percent of married women under 45 were currently practicing contraception (including 10.6 percent who themselves, or their husbands, had been sterilized for contraceptive purposes). Of the remaining 35 percent, most were pregnant, trying to get pregnant, in postpartum, or sterile or subfecund. Among the 5884 then married women surveyed, pills were being used by 22.3 percent and IUDs by 4.8 percent, with similar percentages among both black and whites. These were marked rises from the respective percentages of 15.3 and 0.7 reported five years earlier by 4810 similar women in the 1965 National Fertility Study (266, Table 2). However, the study also revealed that although more recently married U.S. women had become considerably more adept at tailoring their reproduction to their fertility intentions than those married during the 1950s, principally due to adoption of the pill, overall, one-third of couples using contraception during 1966-70 to prevent pregnancy had children anyway (155, 198). Detailed analysis based on reported experience following the first pregnancy revealed that, within their first year of exposure to the risk of unintended conception, 26 percent of couples failed to delay a pregnancy they wanted later and 14 percent failed to prevent a pregnancy they did not intend to have at all (198). Higher failure rates would undoubtedly have been registered had it been possible to collect reliable information on contraceptive and coital experience before the first pregnancy—much of it probably premarital (198). Younger women are much more prone to failure than older women, and blacks than whites. Ryder concluded that, as the 1970s began, substantial numbers of U.S. couples were using ineffective methods of contraception (16 percent used coitus interruptus, foam, rhythm, douche, or "other methods" [266, Table 2]) or were using effective methods carelessly (155).

In the first two years under liberal abortion, 17-18 percent of resident aborters in New York City were under age 20 (231, Table 4). A 1971 nationwide survey by Zelnik and Kantner of 4611 unmarried women aged 15 to 19 disclosed that "pervasive misinformation" existed about the risk of pregnancy, and that among those who have had intercourse by age 20 (54 percent of black women and 23 percent of whites in the total sample; rising to 81 percent and 40 percent respectively among respondents then aged 19) there is a "high degree of risk taking" (273). Of the sexually experienced, about half of these unmarried teenagers of both races had used no contraception during their most recent intercourse. When contraception was used, black women relied more on douching (43 percent) and whites on coitus interruptus (59 percent), and both races relied heavily on condoms. Only a quarter of the young women of both races who used any contraception had used pills most recently.

Tietze and Dawson note that the annual total numbers of known pregnancies (legal abortions plus live births) in New York City during the second year after passage of the abortion act was substantially less than the total of the first year, suggesting that the act had not led to any significant deterioration in contraceptive practice (231, p. 50). On the contrary, contraception probably improved in these years. This is deduced from the fact that legal abortions among New York City residents rose by only 7700 between the first and second full year after the act came into force—from 67,400 to 75,100 (and by a still much less 2800 in the third year [230]). Assuming a "reasonable" level of contraception, this increase of 7700 could avert only about 6400 births (1.2 abortions = 1 live birth in a population presumably practicing effective contraception; see Introduction). Births in 1972 were actually 18,100 fewer than might have been expected on the basis of 1971 fertility rates, so that although there were also 1100 fewer marriages than in the preceding year, the researchers conclude that a large part of the birth drop was due to a significant improvement in contraceptive practice—an improvement that was probably part of an earlier general trend (181, 229).

Substitution of Legal for Illegal Abortion in Hungary, Japan, and New York City and the United States as a Whole

Tietze and Dawson emphasize that "levels and trends of birth rates are determined by broad social forces, the response to which is facilitated by a greater availability of abortion" (231, p. 49). They feel it likely that fertility declines such as noted in Eastern Europe, Japan, and New York City would have been less marked if abortion laws had not been liberalized, but also stress that birth rates would probably have declined to some extent in Eastern Europe in the 1960s and in the United States in the early 1970s even without changes in abortion policy. "These declines would have been achieved by more widespread or more diligent use of contraception and by more frequent illegal abortions."

It will never be known if, for example, contraceptive practice in the United States would have become more diligent in the 1970s than it apparently was at the beginning of the decade had legal abortion not become increasingly available—as it undoubtedly will—although it has been seen that permissive abortion laws probably did somewhat retard adoption of more effective methods, in at least Hungary in the 1960s. Similarly, since numbers of abortions prior to legalization can never be known with certainty it is impossible to measure by how much subsequent legal abortions may outstrip those that might have occurred without law changes and hence have a net impact on subsequent declines in fertility. However, in this vein, it is argued that with respect to at least Hungary and Japan liberalization of abortion had less to do with subsequent fertility declines than it would appear.

Hungary

Potts, Diggory, and Peel point out that in Hungary in 1952 there were 185,000 live births and 1700 legal abortions. Twelve years later and after the alteration of the law there were 184,400 legal abortions, but the number of live births had not fallen correspondingly, and in fact stood at 132,100. Therefore they surmise that criminal abortion must have been common in 1952 and that a significant proportion of the legal abortions in 1964 would have occurred as illegal abortions if the law had remained unchanged (182, Chapter 3).

Similarly, Klinger argues that in Hungary legalization of abortion has not changed the *relative* impact of abortion in fertility control. From 1920 to 1940 completed family size averaged three children–some 3.5 births less than the total pregnancies which Hungarian historical data suggests as a feasible maximum in the absence of fertility control. In 1967 Hungarian completed family size averaged two children. Taking into account lesser use of contraception, Klinger reckons that abortions in the restricted interwar period must have averaged 2 per woman–scarcely less than the estimated lifetime average of 2.6 legal abortions in 1967 (122). However, it should be noted that average actual (and presumably desired) family size in Hungary has declined from three children to two from the pre- to the postabortion legalization period. While the above-noted socioeconomic changes have undoubtedly influenced this, McIntyre also suggests that the availability of safe, inexpensive abortion and subsequent appearance of many one- and two-child families may have had a "demonstration" effect which in itself altered average ideas of what is the "normal" number of children (139).

Japan-Ryukyu Islands

Potts, Diggory, and Peel also note that in the past two decades birth rates in the Ryukyu Islands have paralleled those of their cultural partner, Japan–including the "Fiery Horse" dip (Figure 2-11)–although under U.S. administration from the end of World War II until 1972 abortion was technically illegal in the islands. In the islands, 62 percent of 380 contracepting women reported use of abortion, compared to 65 percent in a similar Japanese survey. The researchers remark that the "inference is that Japan's liberal abortion made visible a broad trend that would have occurred even if the law had never been liberalized." They attribute the higher level (if not the trend) in the fertility of the Ryukyu Islands to economic factors–1971 per capita Gross National Product being U.S. $580 in these islands, compared to U.S. $1190 in Japan (182, Chapter 3).

New York City, and the United States as a Whole

Tietze estimates that some 50,000 illegal abortions must have been obtained annually by New York City residents prior to the 1970 law change; and thus,

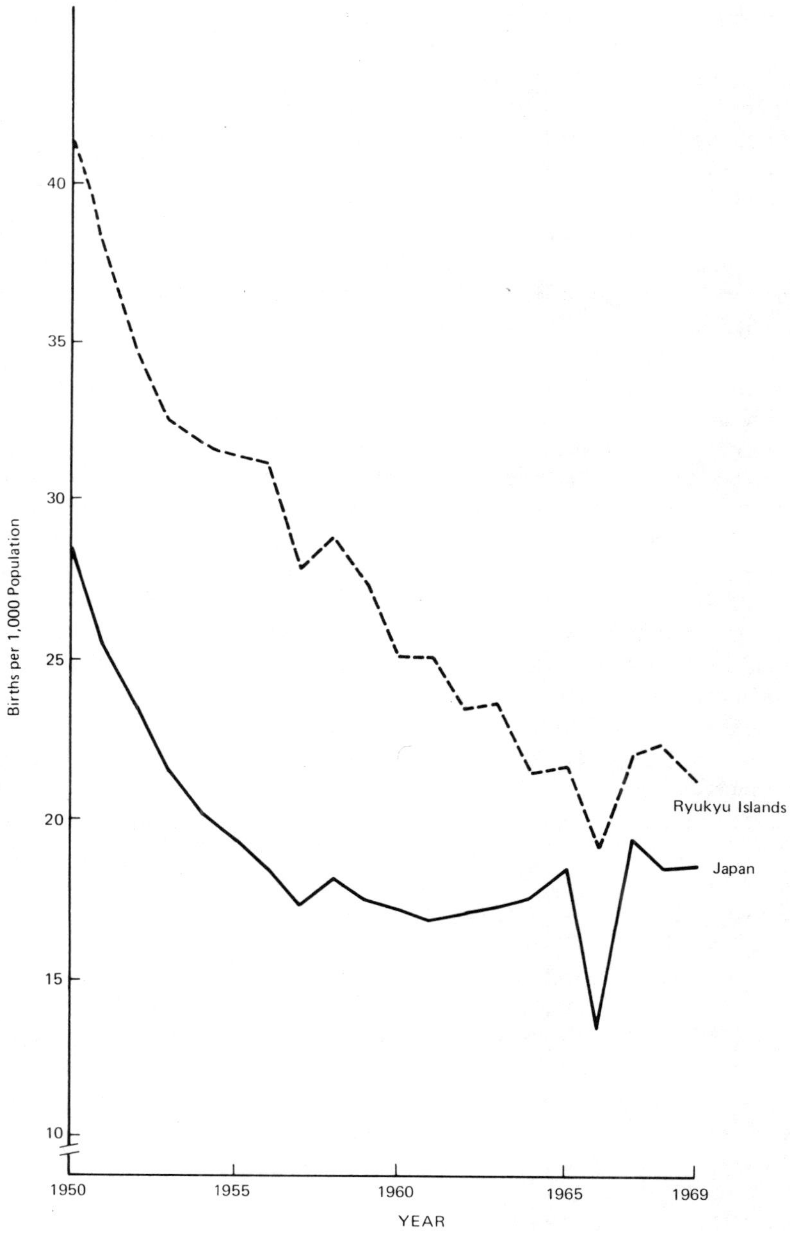

Figure 2-11. Births per 1,000 Population, Japan (Abortion Legal) and the Ryukyu Islands (Abortion Illegal), 1950-69. Source: M. Potts. *IPPF panel of experts on abortion. Tables of Statistics.* London: International Planned Parenthood Federation, 1971, table 44.

only some 25 percent of the 67,400 legal abortions performed on residents in the first year could be taken as responsible for the amount of fertility decline that occurred beyond what might have been expected on the basis of concurrent national trends. Projecting the New York experience to the United States as a whole, Tietze estimated that there would have been a demand for 1,640,000 legal abortions in 1972 had abortion on request then already been available nationwide. This would have dropped births by 410,000, taking about 2.0 points off the 1972 birth rate of 15.6 (228). Tietze considers this a modest potential initial impact, but Berelson remarks that "it may sound light but is substantial when measured against other single impacts in a short period of time" (16, pp. 15-16). Bumpass and Presser observe that "much of this decline in New York City may represent the short-run impact of people who have chosen to delay first births. However, much also represents direct and indirect reductions of total family size and hence has significant implications for the growth of the U.S. population" (29, p. 44).

Tietze expects that the demographic impact of elective abortion would increase over the years in the United States as legal availability and improved delivery services increased acceptance of abortion to the point where all or most unwanted pregnancies would be aborted (228, p. 584). If all U.S. couples were henceforth able to restrict family size to the average 2.5 children reported as wanted in the 1970 National Fertility Study (200), actual completed family size would be little more than 2.1 births per woman (or 2.2 births for the 95 percent of women who now eventually marry in the United States [244]). This is the replacement level fertility that at current mortality rates (and assuming no immigration) would bring the growth of the U.S. population to a halt, after a lag of about seventy years to adjust for currently swollen cohorts of women in, or about to enter, their childbearing years. Replacement level fertility may be even closer to realization in the United States if the youngest women now marrying can restrict completed family size to their current expectations. Women already married at ages 18 to 24 reported in the Census Bureau's Current Population Surveys of June 1972 and June 1973 that they expected an average of 2.3 children (a marked contrast with the average anticipation of 2.9 found for young wives in a 1967 survey and 3.1 in 1965 [245]). Recent past experience suggests that this could result in an average completed family size of 2.1 for all women in the cohort now aged 18 to 24 (244). (In June 1972, nearly half of the 18-24-year-old age group had not yet married. Women marrying later generally have lower completed family sizes than those marrying young.)

Illegal Abortion Following Legalization in Eastern Europe, Japan, and New York City

Sharp declines in abortion-related mortality (231, Table 27) suggest that elective abortion has all but eradicated illegal abortion in *Eastern Europe.* A residual remains, however—e.g., an estimated 5000 illegal abortions in Czechoslovakia in 1968, eleven years after the law was liberalized (33, p. 232)—probably in a desire by some unmarried women to avoid even the minimal administrative procedures required (231, p. 49), and among the small percentage of women whose requests for abortion are denied (213). *Japan* is said to have virtually no illegal abortion today (148). In *New York City*, hospital admissions for treatment of abortion complications declined sharply in 1970-72 (163), and the rate of deaths attributed to all abortions dropped by more than half between 1969 and 1971 (1.42 to 0.69 deaths per 100,000 women aged 15 to 44 [231, Table 27]), which also suggests that the very broad law change of 1970, requiring no official intervention, significantly reduced numbers of illegal abortions.

People's Republic of China

Tietze and Dawson point out that the "People's Republic of China is the only example of a country with a traditionally high birth rate . . . where abortion on request has been made available not only *de jure* but apparently *de facto* as well" (231, p. 49). China has had three successive and vigorous birth-control campaigns, stressing late marriage and no more than two planned, well-spaced births: 1956 to 1958, 1962 to 1966, and 1969 to the present, with interruptions due to the "Great Leap Forward" and the "Cultural Revolution" (6). Abortion was first made available in 1957 and is currently included as part of the national family program (which at the beginning of 1974 was the case nowhere else except in Tunisia). Like all contraceptive and medical services, it is free and, moreover, entitles a working woman to fifteen days' paid leave (72). (At least three other high-birth-rate countries had technically legalized abortion on broad terms by early 1974. In 1965, *Tunisia* authorized abortion on request within the national family planning program for any woman with at least five living children. Legal abortions performed within the national family planning program numbered only 2700 in 1970 [58] , but in 1971, 13,000 legal abortions were performed in all institutions under the Ministry of Health [241] —amounting to 7 percent of live births in that year, compared to 12 percent among residents of England and Wales in the same year [58] . A recent decline in the birth rate to below 40 per 1000 population is attributed largely to rising ages at marriage and somewhat to inauguration of the national family planning program in 1966 [128] . Elective abortion in the first trimester of pregnancy for any woman was legalized in September 1973 [234] , a move officially acknowledged as one effort to accelerate fertility declines. *India's* 1971 Medical Termination of Pregnancy Act, effective April 1972, permits termination of any pregnancy in a married woman claimed as due to contraceptive failure [105] . Implementation of the act has been slow, especially in rural areas, and the number of legal abortions performed is apparently still small, at least when compared to the estimated annual total of at least 4 million illegal abortions [231, 260] . *Zambia* legalized abortion in 1972 along the lines of the British act of 1967, but no data have been issued to date. The birth rate is estimated as still nearly 50 per 1000 [240]. *Iran*, with an estimated 1965-70 annual birth rate of 45.4 per 1000 [239], is scheduled to legalize abortion on broad terms in August 1974 [230]. Another "developing" state, *Singapore*, already had a birth rate in the low 20s per 1000 at the time of abortion liberalization in 1970 [see Chapter 4].)

Vacuum aspiration was invented and perfected in China, and according to Faundes and Luukkainen, following a March 1972 visit, is practiced by "barefoot doctors" and midwives in rural areas and nurses in urban areas (72). Chen reports, however, after a visit later in 1972, that barefoot doctors serve only as referral points for abortions, which are then performed by qualified physicians, although a recently issued "retraining" manual for barefoot doctors suggests that such paramedical personnel will increasingly be trained to perform abortions (40).

Officially, abortion has been promoted only as a backstop to contraceptive failure, rather than as a primary means for family control (74). No official statistics on its incidence have ever been released. Recent visitors feel it is now being displaced by pills, IUDs, and sterilization, but that it is still widespread (40, 72). Thus it appears that abortion has been an important factor in the apparent decline of the population growth rate to below 2 percent annually since about 1966 (40), which Potts, Diggory, and Peel claim is a "remarkable achievement equalled by no other country in a similar state of development" (182, Chapter 3). (For 1965-70, the U.N. estimates an average annual birth rate of 33.1 per 1000 for the People's Republic of China, compared to, for instance, 42.8 for India [240].) However, Tietze and Dawson caution that "whether the addition of elective abortion to ongoing family planning programs in other countries would result in similar declines, without a restructuring of the entire society, such as has taken place in China, is not known" (231, p. 49). In a May 1972 report to the Joint Economic Committee of the U.S. Congress, Aird is skeptical of published reports to that date of urban birth rates as low as 6 per 1000 and rural rates of 18-20 per 1000, in view of the long-entrenched Chinese desire for sons and large families, and also doubts reports of rising ages at marriage in response to the officially recommended 23 for women and 26 for men, "accompanied by strictly observed chastity prior to marriage." In addition, he comments that although "abortions and sterilizations may number in the tens of thousands annually, [they] scarcely constitute a perceptible reduction in the annual cohort of over 30 million births" (6, p. 317). However, later reports by actual visitors to China, such as Chen, Faundes and Luukkainen, and Katagiri, persist in reports of such late marriage, premarital chastity, and declining birth rates (40, 72, 117).

3 Fertility Trends Following Restriction of Permissive Abortion

Official restriction of legal abortion has only a temporary effect on birth rates where a small-family ideal is entrenched.

Official alarm at declining birth rates and soaring abortion rates prompted restrictions of legal abortion in Czechoslovakia in late 1962, Romania in October 1966, and Bulgaria in 1968, 1972, and 1973 (as well as in the U.S.S.R. from 1936 to 1955).[a] These restrictions were relatively mild in *Czechoslovakia*, involving mainly childless women and reintroduction of abortion fees, and were again relaxed in 1966 (54). (Stricter administrative procedures for granting abortions were again ordered by the Czechoslovakian government in May 1973 [53].) In *Romania*, where abortions had risen to the record level of four per live birth in 1965, the restrictions were abrupt and by Eastern European standards relatively drastic, limiting abortion to cases involving risk to the mother's life or of congenital malformation, rape, women over 45 or supporting four living children, and an explicitly defined set of physical and mental conditions (191, 224). *Bulgaria's* recent series of restrictions still permits abortion on request to unmarried women and married women with two or more living children who press their case (28). At the same time in all three countries pronatalist incentives were introduced or strengthened—maternity leaves extended, family allowances increased, third births particularly compensated, larger families granted access to apartments and tax reductions, etc. In Romania, a childlessness tax on persons aged over 25 was reintroduced, divorce sharply curtailed, and official importation of pills and IUDs discontinued (60).

Figure 3-1 portrays *ensuing birth-rate trends*. In all cases there is an immediate annual rise in birth rates; most dramatically in Romania, where the rise was from a low of 12.8 per 1000 in December 1966 (one month after the new law took effect) to 39.9 in September 1967. But in each case the increase was shortlasting, and with no change in abortion restrictions, birth rates resumed downward trends (dropping back to 18.8 in Romania by 1972 [58]), probably through use of traditional contraceptive methods, clandestine purchase of modern contraceptives (in Romania), resort to illegal abortions, and reduced probability of conception for a period of time after childbirth (60, 214).

[a]As of January 1974, Hungary has withdrawn unrestricted abortion on request for married women with fewer than two living children or those with two children who have not previously had an abortion, tightened administrative procedures, and raised abortion fees (103).

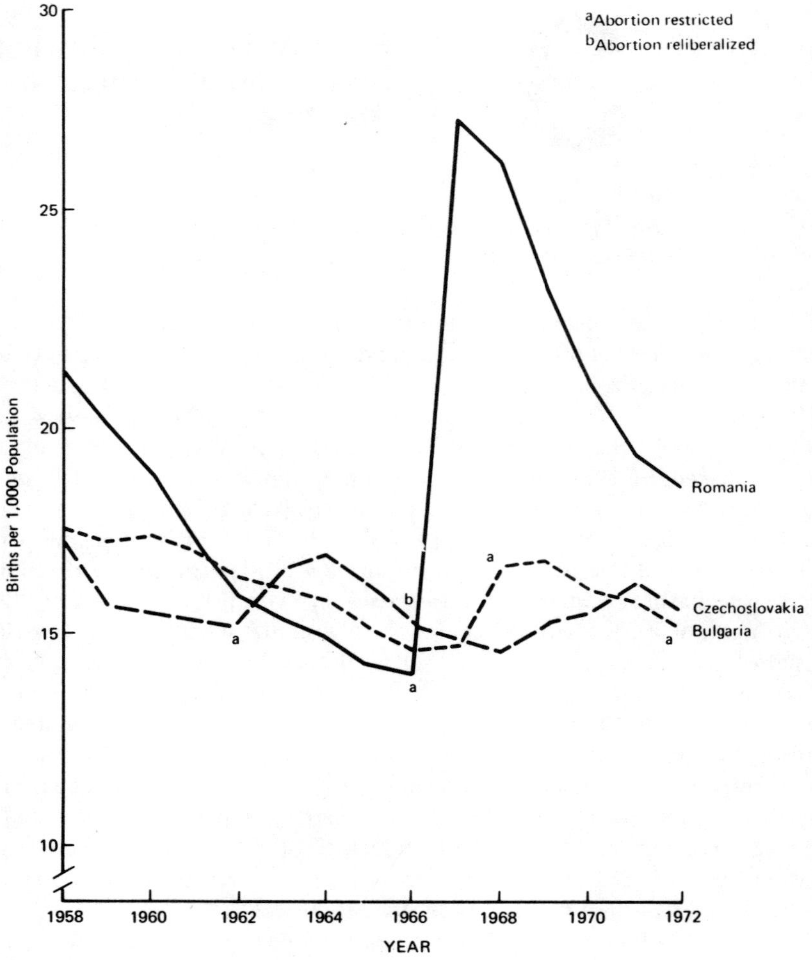

Figure 3-1. Birth Rates Associated with Deliberalization of Abortion plus Deliberate Pronatalist Policies, Bulgaria, Czechoslovakia, Romania, 1958-72. Source: H.P. David, M.G. Kalis, and C. Tietze. *Selected abortion statistics: an international summary.* Washington: AIR/Transnational Family Research Institute, 1973 (birth rates updated as reported to March 1974).

4 Trends Following More Moderate Extension of Legal Abortion

More gradual decline in birth rates is noted where change is from restrictive to moderate legal status of abortion (33, p. 291).

Scandinavia

Abortion Liberalization–De Jure and De Facto

The Nordic countries were among the first to liberalize abortion laws, with first steps taken in Iceland, Sweden, and Denmark in the 1930s. Laws were further liberalized in Sweden in 1946 and 1963, and in Denmark in 1956, 1970, and 1973. Finland's liberalized abortion statute of 1950 was revised in 1970. The 1960 liberal abortion statute of Norway, effective in 1963, merely codified what had long been accepted medical practice (62, 63, 64, 77, 78, 158, 219, 226, 231).

Until the recent revisions in Denmark and Finland, the range of permissible indications included: medical (physical or mental illness makes the pregnancy and childbirth a serious threat to the woman's health); humanitarian (pregnancy as a result of rape or incest or in a woman under a certain age); and eugenic (danger of fetal abnormality) (3). A fourth mixed sociomedical indication provided that existing or potential physical and mental health hazards presented by the woman's present and foreseeable future living conditions also be taken into account in making the decision (3, 226). In 1970, Denmark and Finland legalized abortion on request for women aged at least 38 (Denmark) or 40 (Finland), with four children already born (Finland) or aged under 18 living at home (Denmark), and, in the case of Finland, if conception occurred under age 17. For other abortions the range was broadened to include the first purely *social* indications, without reference to the woman's health, recognized in Scandinavia, particularly youth and immaturity in Denmark and unmarried status or unfinished education in Finland (114, 130, 231). In the words of the 1970 Danish law: "In reaching the decision, consideration shall be paid to the woman's age, the effort involved in her occupation, and her personal circumstances in other respects, as well as the circumstances of the family from the point of view of housing, income, and health." In October 1973 the Danish law was extended to permit abortion at any woman's request during the first trimester of pregnancy (64).

Motives behind the laws and subsequent revisions have been multiple. While it was agreed that in the interest of the woman the danger and expense of illegal abortions should be combated by reasonably liberal legislation, on the other hand the area's already low birth rates (only Finland's being over 20 per 1000 population by 1950) dictated that in the interest of society pregnancies should be carried to term whenever possible (159). Thus all the countries have made their abortion laws part of a general effort to assist pregnant women—those who want their child and those who do not (33, p. 190)—with counseling and assistance freely available (also for contraception), free antenatal, hospital, and postnatal care, dental grants, housing allowances, and generous maternity grants for the wed and unwed alike (23, 218).

Until the early 1960s the laws were interpreted with caution, and administrative procedures were generally elaborate. Up to 1965 in Sweden, more than 85 percent of all legal abortions required authorization by the National Board of Health in Stockholm, with decisions based on written reports from physicians examining women seeking abortion. The remaining 15 percent were performed on the authority of a certificate signed by two physicians. In Denmark all but the 10 percent of abortions granted on medical grounds required the unanimous authorization of a committee comprised of a psychiatrist, a gynecologist, and a social worker, attached to the local Mother's Aid, a publicly supported organization which conducts a thorough medical and social investigation. In Finland and Norway the administrative machinery has been relatively decentralized, with most legal abortions approved by two physicians (226).

Bureaucratic delays resulted in a higher proportion of second trimester abortions and consequently higher rates of abortion complications and mortality than in Eastern Europe and Japan. Since 1965 growing public dissatisfaction with such delays and comparatively strict eligibility requirements has led to an increasing permissiveness in interpretation and application of abortion laws and the recent Danish and Finnish revisions. Sweden has debated abortion on request for a number of years but no decision has been taken (231). However, by 1970 three out of five abortions were being granted by the less time-consuming two-physician procedure; numbers of applicants increased, and by 1972, 96 percent of all applications were being approved, compared to 62 percent in 1960 (55, 231). Similarly in Denmark there was a steady rise in the number of applications and in the percentage of applications approved (33). In 1971-72, 91 percent of requests for abortions brought to Mother's Aid centers were approved (258).

Ensuing Levels of Legal Abortion and Concurrent Birth Trends

Levels of legal abortion in Scandinavia have clearly reflected the progressive liberalization and interpretation of the law. In the pre-1960 restrictive period no country registered more than 5800 in any one year (58). At their pre-1960 peak in Sweden, for instance, 1951, legal abortions terminated less than 6 percent of all pregnancies and this proportion declined to under 3 percent in 1960 (79), resulting in a legal abortion rate far below that of the crude birth rate (Figure 4-1). In 1960, the highest ratio of legal abortions to live births was that of Finland, at 75 (Table 4-1). In that year the comparable ratio stood at 662 in Japan and 1108 in Hungary (58). Concurrently, birth rates fell by no more than 10 percent from the level of the early 1950s, except for Finland, whose 1950-54 average birth rate of 23 per 1000 population was higher than the 16-19 range of the other three countries (Figure 4-2).

With increasing de facto liberalization after 1965, numbers of legal abortions and legal abortion ratios and rates climbed steeply (Table 4-1, and Figure 4-1 for Sweden). Concomitantly, until 1970, birth rates fell at a steeper rate than in the 1950s, after an upturn from 1960 to 1965 (Figure 4-2). For Sweden, Svala and Ottosson suggest that the 1965-70 fertility drop may be partially explained by the increase in legal abortions, although improved contraception (below) is probably equally if not more important (161, 218). By complicated calculations

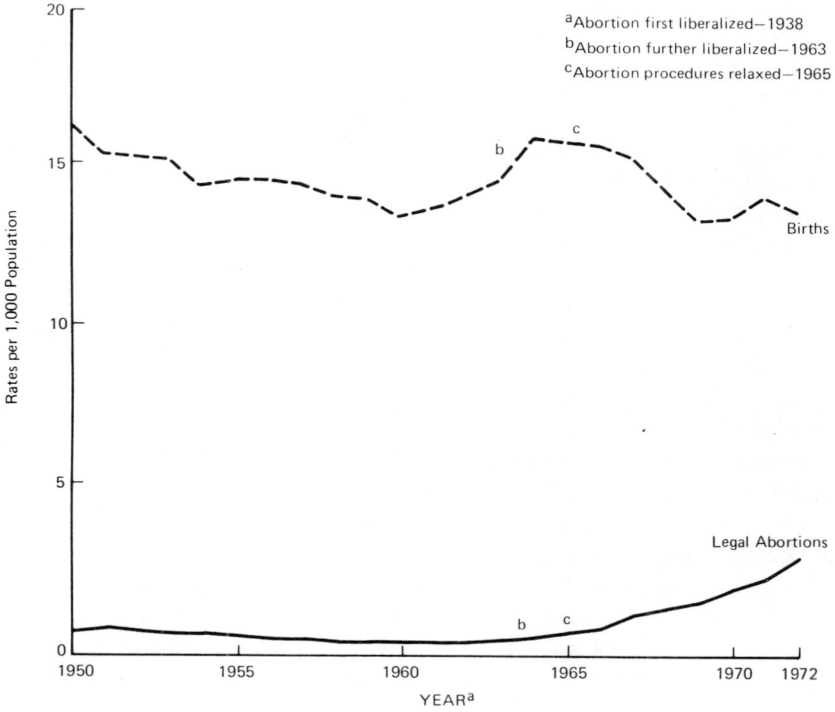

Figure 4-1. Births and Legal Abortions per 1,000 Population, Sweden, 1950-72. Source: Same as Figure 3-1.

Table 4-1
Numbers and Ratios of Legal Abortions, and Birth Rates, Denmark, Finland, Norway, and Sweden, Selected Years, 1960-72

	Denmark[a]			Finland[b]		
Year	Number of Legal Abortions	Legal Abortions per 1,000 Live Births	Live Births per 1,000 Population	Number of Legal Abortions	Legal Abortions per 1,000 Live Births	Live Births per 1,000 Population
1960	3,900	52	16.6	6,200	75	18.5
1965	5,200	61	18.0	4,800	61	16.9
1967	6,300	78	16.8	5,600	73	16.6
1969	7,500 (1969-70)	89	14.6	8,200	121	14.3
1970	10,100 (1970-71)	106	14.4	14,800	229	13.7
1971	11,500 (1971-72)	133	15.2	20,400	332	13.1
1972		152	15.2			12.7

Source: H.P. David, M.G. Kalis, and C. Tietze, *Selected abortion statistics: An international summary.* Washington: AIR/Transnational Family Research Institute, January 1973, with updating of statistics as reported to March 1974.

[a]Abortion law liberalized 1937, 1956, 1970 (April 1), 1973 (October. On request).

of the impact of legal abortion and IUD and pill use on projections of previous population trends, Sjovall concludes that the increase in legal abortion was responsible for the 1964-69 fertility drop mostly among oldest (40 to 44) and youngest (15 to 19) women. Among women aged 35 to 39 it was as important as IUDs or pills in averting births, but "only to a small extent" accountable for fertility declines among the intermediate group aged 20 to 34 (208). Ottosson has produced the following figure for Sweden (Figure 4-3) which suggests that the rise and fall in abortion ratios has been at least to some degree mirrored by trends in the net reproduction rate, especially since 1965. (The net reproduction rate represents the average number of daughters that a cohort of newborn girl babies would bear if they were exposed up to the end of their reproductive life to a fixed schedule of fertility and mortality rates, which in this case were those prevailing in Sweden in each of the years covered in Figure 4-3.)

The slight 1970-71 upturn in birth rates in Denmark, Norway, and Sweden (although slightly down again the following year in the latter two) may be due in part to the entry into childbearing ages of the comparatively swollen cohorts of 1945-49, when birth rates rose to 22 in Denmark, 21 in Norway, and 19 in Sweden. However, Finland's birth rate of that period was highest at 27 (240). In contrast to the other three countries, its birth rate dropped sharply from 1970 to 1971, following the abortion law change of June 1970 (114). In 1971 its

Norway[c]			Sweden[d]		
Number of Legal Abortions	Legal Abortions per 1,000 Live Births	Live Births per 1,000 Population	Number of Legal Abortions	Legal Abortions per 1,000 Live Births	Live Births per 1,000 Population
		17.3	2,800	27	13.7
3,400	51	17.8	6,200	51	15.9
5,000	75	17.6	9,700	80	15.4
6,300	93	17.6	13,700	128	13.5
7,800	121	16.5	16,100	146	13.6
10,200	155	16.8	19,300	169	14.1
12,200	187	16.6	24,200	216	13.8

[b]Abortion law liberalized 1950, 1970 (June 1).

[c]Abortion law liberalized 1960, implemented 1963.

[d]Abortion law liberalized 1938, 1963.

birth rate of 13 per 1000 was lowest and its abortion ratio of 332 highest in Scandinavia. Following the similar 1970 abortion law revisions, numbers of legal abortions in Finland jumped by 80 percent, from 8200 in 1969 to 14,800 in 1970, while in Denmark legal abortions rose by just over a third–from 7500 in the twelve months preceding the April 1970 law change to 10,100 in the twelve succeeding months (Table 4-1). It should be noted that legal abortions also increased substantially in Sweden and Norway with no law changes.

Numbers of *out-of-wedlock births* climbed sharply in Sweden during the 1960s, despite high proportions of unmarried women among legal aborters (57 percent in 1970 [231, Table 9]), and an abortion rate for women under 20 which by 1968 was highest of any age group (13 per 1000 in 1970, compared to 12 per 1000 among women aged 20 to 24, the next highest group [231, Table 5]). By 1969, out-of-wedlock births comprised 16.2 percent of all births (218), compared to 5.5 percent among white U.S. women in that year (250). The word "illegitimate" was erased from Swedish statute books in 1917, and out-of-wedlock children have all the legal and social rights of those born within marriage (218). Unwed motherhood is similarly tolerated in Denmark (258), although perhaps slightly less common–10.2 percent of all births in 1966 (last year for which data are available), compared to 14.6 percent in Sweden in the same year (240: 1969, Table 21). Until the late 1960s, Denmark and Finland

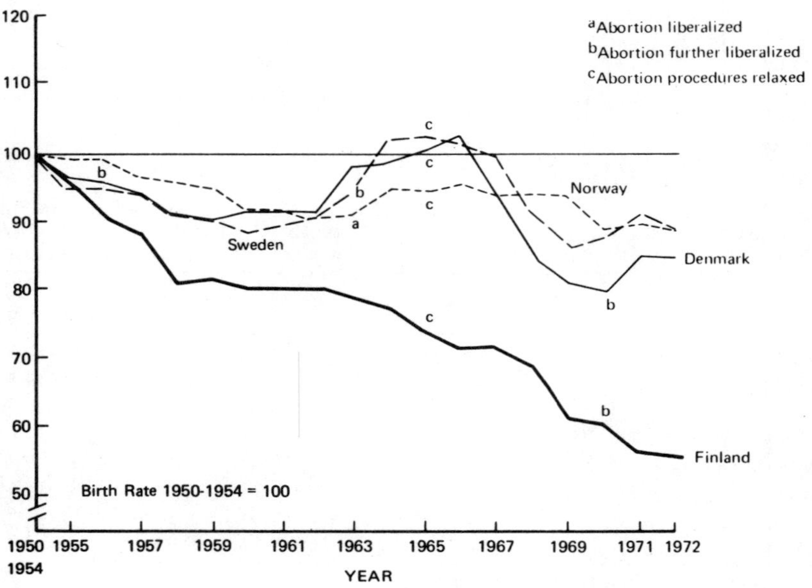

Figure 4-2. Birth Trends in Denmark, Finland, Norway, and Sweden, 1950-54 to 1972. Source: Patterned after similar figures in A.R. Omran. Abortion in the demographic transition. In R. Revelle (ed.), *Rapid population growth: Consequences and policy implications.* Vol. 2. Baltimore: The Johns Hopkins Press, 1971, figure 7, p. 523. Derived from basic data given in United Nations, Statistical Office. *Demographic yearbooks.* New York: Author, various years; United Nations, Statistical Office. *Population and vital statistics report: Data available as of 1 October 1973.* New York: Author, Statistical Papers, Series A, Vol. 25, Nos. 3 and 4, 1973.

had lesser proportions of unmarried women among legal aborters than Sweden—about 40 percent each, in contrast to Sweden's 56 percent in 1969 (231, Table 9). Finland and Norway have also had considerably smaller proportions of out-of-wedlock births than the other two Scandinavian countries—no more than 5 to 6 percent by the late 1960s (18, 240: 1969, Table 21).

Concomitant Contraceptive Use

No contraceptive information is available for Norway and Finland. Presumably there, too, pills and IUDs are on the increase as in *Sweden* (although Finland's

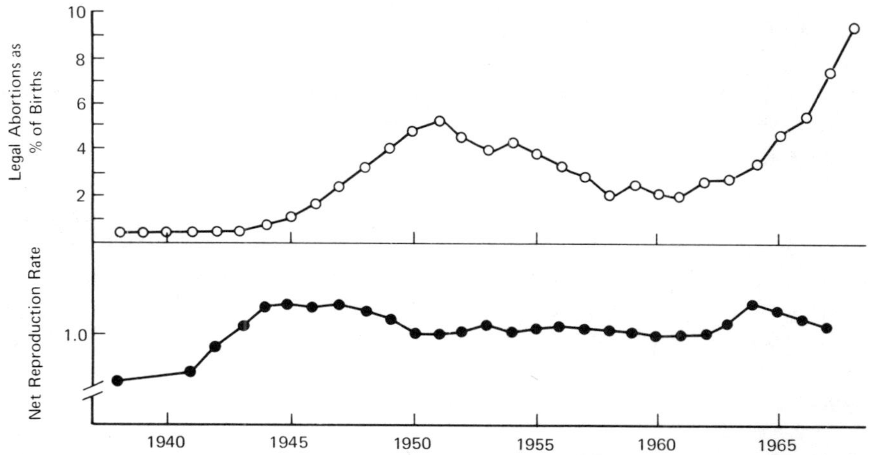

Figure 4-3. Legal Abortions in Relation to Number of Births and Net Reproduction Rate, Sweden, 1938-67. Source: Reprinted with permission of Blackwell Scientific Publications, Ltd. from J.O. Ottosson. Legal abortion in Sweden: Thirty years' experience. *Journal of Biosocial Science*, 1971, 3, text-figure 2, p. 177. Note: The pattern of successive peaking of the *legal* abortion ratio in Sweden, seen in this figure, suggests that abortion use may not necessarily peak only once in the course of a country's demographic transition, as implied in the Requena-Klinger model (figure 1-1). In some cases, swells and troughs in abortion incidence may occur in response to fluctuations in official permissiveness (see text), although in Sweden the *total* incidence of abortion (legal and illegal) possibly changed little in these 30 years (see text). Also, of course, the country has long been near or at the end of its demographic transition.

recent upsurge of abortions suggests otherwise). Pills were introduced to Sweden in 1964; IUDs in 1966 (208). In a 1967 survey only 14 percent of respondents reported use of the pill during their latest intercourse, but by 1972 the Swedish Family Planning Association estimated pill use by 28 percent of women aged 15 to 44—about 450,000 women—with another some 30,000 using IUDs (55, 218). (In the United States in 1970, an estimated 22 percent of married women were on the pill, and by the end of 1971, 18 percent of all British women of childbearing age were.) The Swedish health system provides abortions free, but until recently contraceptives have not been reimbursable. Pills and IUDs must be prescribed by a physician after examination, which costs about $20 privately or requires a long wait for an appointment at one of the few public family planning centers or only two centers run by the Family Planning Association (55).

Sterilization is still illegal for contraceptive purposes. In the 1967 survey, 17 percent reported use of coitus interruptus, while the most commonly used contraceptive was the condom—38 percent. In Sweden condoms are widely advertised and available—from coin-operated dispensers at supermarket checkout counters, for example. Sex education is required in all schools from earliest years (55).

In *Denmark*, survey data on contraceptive use are available only for Copenhagen, indicating that no contraception was used by two-thirds of a cross-section of married housewives in 1952, but that this had dropped to 26 percent in 1959 and 19 percent in 1968 among mothers aged under 21 (24). By 1968, pills were used by 43 percent of married mothers under 21, and 21 percent of the unmarried, and IUDs by 6 percent of both, with condom use reported by 34 and 8 percent respectively.

Substitution of Legal for Illegal Abortion in Sweden, Denmark, and Finland

In *Sweden*, the abortion law, as written and practiced, appears to have had a relatively small net impact on *long-term* fertility trends. About 1970, the birth rate averaged 13.5 to 13.6—little lower than the average 14.5 per 1000 population of the early 1930s which touched off a public clamor concerning a population crisis, precipitated by the famous Myrdal report of 1934 (153). Potts, Diggory, and Peel point out that in that period, before the first abortion law change of 1938, numbers of illegal abortions were estimated at 10,000 to 20,000 annually, or 100 to 200 induced abortions per 1000 live births—levels comparable to those observed for legal abortions in the most recent years (Table 4-1; although 24,200 were recorded for 1972, 216 per 1000 live births), more than thirty years after the first law change. Since contraceptive practice has improved meanwhile, the total number of induced abortions might be expected to have declined. They suggest that the main results of the progressively more liberal legal abortion situation have been a significant transfer from illegal to legal abortions (according to Ohrberg, illegal abortions by 1969 were "no longer a numerical problem" [159]), possibly a decline in the total number (illegal and legal) of abortions among the married, and an increase in the number of premarital pregnancies and abortion rates among the young unmarried (182, Chapter 3).

For *Denmark*, recent research suggests that the April 1970 abortion liberalization resulted in more than a simple replacement of illegal with legal abortions. Sele and Norgaard (204) estimate illegal abortions as about 6000 nationally in 1960 (in contrast to 10,000 estimated by Wagner and Wagner [258]), when registered legal abortions totaled 3900 (58). This would yield a total of about 129 abortions (legal plus estimated illegal) per 1000 of the live births in 1960 (77,000). In the twelve months following the April 1970 law change, 10,100 legal abortions were recorded, and Sele and Norgaard estimate that illegal abortions had declined to about 2300 nationwide, yielding a comparable ratio of 163 total abortions per 1000 of the 76,000 births in 1971 (which would be those most affected by abortions in this period). However, total births and birth rates also rose in 1971 (Table 4-1 and Figure 4-2), suggesting that the swell in abortions was not sufficient to offset increased numbers of women in childbearing ages (above) or transient changes in fertility behavior. Nevertheless, Denmark's birth rate of 15 in 1971 was somewhat lower than the average 18 per 1000 of the 1930s. It remains to be seen what fertility trends may be associated with the legalization of abortion on request in October 1973.

In *Finland*, contrary to Denmark's experience, the sharp and continuing increase in legal abortions following the 1970 law change was at least initially accompanied by no decrease in the incidence of illegal abortion, according to Jarvinen (114). This suggests that the law change was indeed an important factor in the associated sharp drop in birth rates—to a regional low of 12.7 in 1972 (two-thirds of the average 20 per 1000 of the 1930s)—although Finnish birth rates had been declining more rapidly than those of the other three countries in the preceding period (Figure 4-2). Berent and Festy have shown that changes in the age, sex, and marital components of Finland's population tended to offset each other with regard to their potential impact on fertility trends from 1950 to 1970, so that actual marital fertility fell as rapidly as crude birth rates to 1965 (10-15 percent decline in both rates in each five-year period), and even more rapidly from 1965 to 1970 (22 percent decline in marital fertility rates compared to 15 percent in crude birth rates [18]).

Scandinavia's well-known high and rising levels of industrialization, urbanization, per capita income, education, and women's labor force participation, and record low rates of infant mortality (see Appendix table for Denmark and Sweden) have resulted in a long-time generally *low desired family size*, e.g., an average of 2.4 children in a recent Swedish survey—above actual completed family size (274). Over the long run, abortion has probably played an important, if diminishing, role in achieving this goal, and will continue to be important as a backstop to contraceptive failure, or nonuse, especially among young, unmarried women. However, it seems that, with the possible exception of Finland, Scandinavia's style of gradually more liberal legal abortion has been more important as a health measure than as a major influence on fertility trends, although short-term fluctuations in fertility appear to be associated with changes in abortion laws or practice in some cases.

Great Britain

Abortion Liberalization—De Jure and De Facto

In Great Britain, the "ferocious" terms of the 1861 Offences Against the Person Act, which made abortion under any circumstances punishable by life imprisonment, were eased somewhat by court rulings of 1938 and 1948 (*Rex vs. Bourne* and *Rex vs. Bermann*), permitting legal termination of pregnancies that posed a serious threat to the life or health of women (167). However, the British medical profession took a conservative attitude toward making use of these rulings (226). The new Abortion Act of October 1967 (effective April 27, 1968), passed "against a background of immense public and parliamentary controversy" (167), was "a recognition by the community that the occurrence of illegal abortion had reached such a level that it posed a serious problem in terms of maternal mortality and morbidity and a racket with implications of 'one law for the rich and another for the poor' " (26).

While similar to the Scandinavian model of the time, the new British law anticipated the 1970 Danish and Finnish changes in authorizing abortion on the certification by two physicians that continuance of the pregnancy would involve injury to the physical or mental health of any existing children of the pregnant woman "greater than if the pregnancy were terminated" (235). As in Scandinavia, a woman's "total environment" may be taken into account in making the decision. Inclusion of this so-called "social" clause caused most controversy at the time of the act's passage, but in practice about 75 percent of legal abortions in the first three years were registered as on grounds of risk to the health of the pregnant woman, and only 15-20 percent on that of existing children (although the latter was a contributing factor in 32 percent of abortions granted to married women in 1970 [109, 205]). It is suggested that the medical profession interpreted "social problems" in traditional medical terms (180). A national opinion poll of January 1970 revealed 61 percent in favor of the "family-environmental" clause of the act (146, Chapter 5).

The act stipulates that abortion be carried out in a hospital or nursing home approved by the Department of Health and Social Security, which in early 1974 still required every woman to remain overnight after the operation (179). (General anesthesia is nearly universal and delays for operating-room space common (180).) However, the act did not lay an obligation upon the National Health Service to provide facilities, and included a conscience clause. To receive a free abortion under the National Health Service, a British resident must first be referred by a general practitioner and then accepted by a consultant gynecologist attached to the NHS hospital in her area. In the first years following the act's implementation, distinct regional variations were noted in the rate of terminations under the National Health Service, with high rates in, for example, London and Newcastle, and low rates in the Midlands—attributed to the uneven distribution of facilities and approving medical professionals (38, 179, 197). A 1970 study disclosed that regional NHS abortion rates were correlated negatively with proportions of general practitioners with conscientious objections and the proportion of their NHS referrals that were rejected (38).

The proportion of NHS hospital abortions among all legal abortions performed on British women declined from 69 to 59 percent between 1969 and

1971 (109). Women refused an NHS abortion can seek a private one. Until 1970 these were only available in private, noncharitable clinics which quickly sprang up to meet the demand, particularly from increasing numbers of foreign women—the act carries no residency requirements—where prices were sometimes extreme (179). However, since 1970, the British (formerly Birmingham) and London Pregnancy Advisory Services have provided an increasing number of abortions in nursing homes which they own (or control strictly) at minimum economic prices, ranging from about U.S. $135 to U.S. $210 for a first-trimester procedure, or on interest-free loans or outright grants (20, 179). (These prices are comparable to those charged by New York City freestanding clinics in 1970-72 for first-trimester abortions, which is surprising in view of lower living costs in Britain. However, first-trimester abortions in the United States are now generally done on an outpatient basis, while an overnight stay is still required in Britain.) In 1972, these services arranged some 30,000 such low-cost abortions—nearly one-third of the 100,000 private abortions in England and Wales in that year (206).

Ensuing Levels of Legal Abortions

Numbers of legal abortions performed on residents of England and Wales rose from an estimated 27,200 in 1967 (67) (the last full year before the new act took effect) to 49,800 in 1969, the first full year after its implementation, 94,600 in 1971, and 108,600 in 1972 (58). In Scotland, the rise among residents was from 3600 in 1969 to 7600 in 1972 (58). (The act does not apply to Northern Ireland.) That this rate of increase was unanticipated seems implicit in the following observation on statistics concerning the first year of implementation: "Thirty-eight thousand abortions [total for all Britain, including nonresidents, in 1968] represent a mere 4½ percent of total live births, and if the figure rises, in subsequent years, to 50,000 or even 60,000 the effect on the birth rate is likely to be small" (167, p. 3). By 1972 in England and Wales alone the 108,600 legal abortions among residents amounted to 15.0 percent of total live births (compared to 21.6 percent in Sweden and 117.0 percent in Hungary in that year), while the 156,700 legal abortions among residents and nonresidents alike represented 21.7 percent of live births (58). However, by 1972 legal abortions to residents still fell more than 12 points short of births per 1000 population (Figure 4-4).

Ensuing Fertility Trends

Figure 4-4 depicts the trends since 1962 in crude birth rates and legal abortion rates per 1000 (resident) population in England and Wales. England and Wales

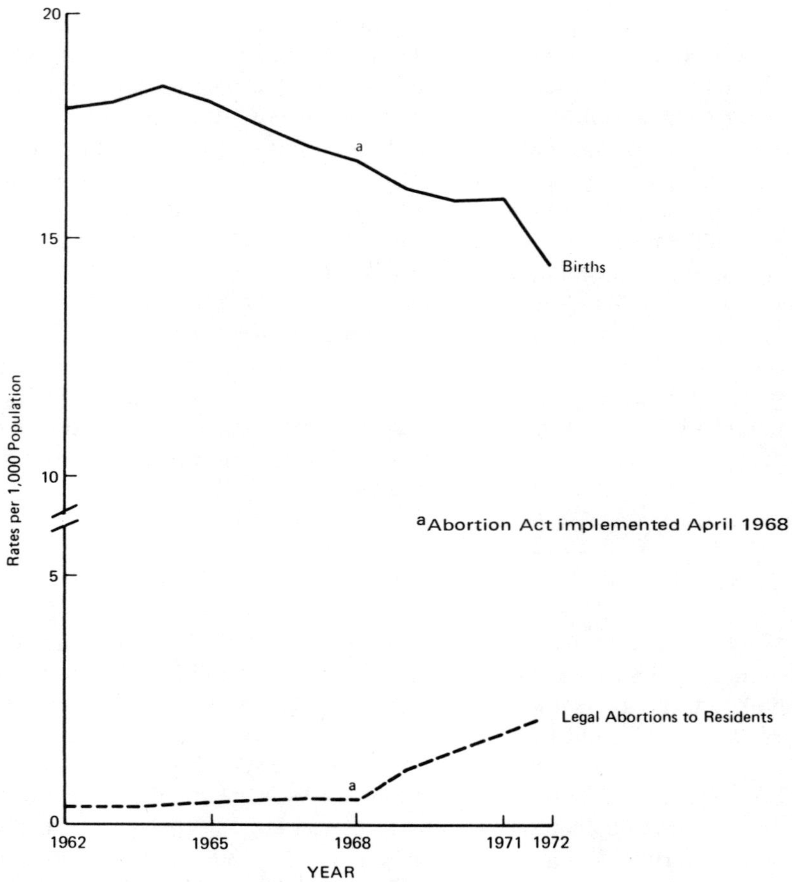

Figure 4-4. Births and Legal Abortions per 1,000 Population, England and Wales, 1962-72. Source: Same as Figure 3-1.

experienced a brief baby boom in 1946 and 1947 (birth rates of 19.2 and 20.5 compared to 14-15 per 1000 during the 1930s [21]), and the "excess" girls of those years—now well into their childbearing years—would tend to inflate the crude birth rate. Figure 4-5 of trends in the general fertility rate (births per 1000 women aged 15 to 44) gives a clearer picture of fertility trends in recent years. Although the fertility rate had been declining from the 1964 peak (probably due to increased use of contraceptives and introduction of the pill—see below), it would seem that the trend line of decrease has accelerated since implementation of the abortion act on April 27, 1968. In addition, as recorded following recent abortion law changes in New York City and in at least three U.S. states (below), there has been a reversal in the long-standing rise of *out-of-wedlock births.*

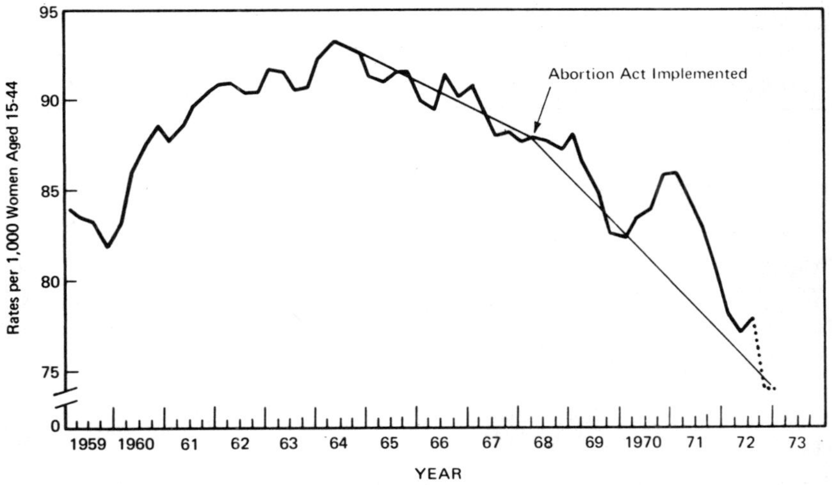

Figure 4-5. General Fertility Rates per 1,000 Women aged 15-44, England and Wales, 1959-73. Source: United Kingdom, Office of Population Censuses and Surveys. *The Registrar General's Quarterly Return for England and Wales, Quarter ended 31 March, 1973.* London: Her Majesty's Stationery Office, 1973, diagram for table 2a, p. 8.

Table 4-2 shows that illegitimate births in England and Wales peaked at 17,600 in the first quarter of 1969—eight to eleven months after the abortion law came into effect—and declined to about 15,800 by the third quarter of 1972, with some fluctuations. The final total of 62,500 illegitimate births in 1972 was 11 percent below the peak of 69,900 in 1967, the last full year before the abortion act became operative. From 1968 to 1971, unwed women made up about 55 percent of all legal aborters in England and Wales (231, Table 9). In the 1970 study already mentioned, greater declines in the rate of out-of-wedlock births (and the proportion of high parity births) from 1967 to 1969 were noted in hospital regions with higher abortion rates (38).

In 1969 there was also a decline for the first time since 1955 in the number of *premaritally conceived births.* From a peak of 74,500 in 1968, births occurring less than eight months after first marriage dropped to 72,600 in 1969 and 67,700 by 1971. The proportion of all live births conceived extramaritally (out-of-wedlock plus premaritally conceived births), which had climbed steadily from 11.1 percent in 1955 to 17.6 percent in 1968, dropped to 17.5 percent in 1969 and 17.0 percent by 1971 (237). The drop would have been more notable had there not been a concomitant decline in total births.

Table 4-2
Numbers *(in Thousands)* of Illegitimate Live Births, by Quarter, Seasonally Adjusted, England and Wales, 1959-72

	Quarter			
Year	First	Second	Third	Fourth
1959	9.5	9.5	9.6	9.5
1960	10.1	10.5	10.9	11.2
1961	11.4	11.8	12.3	13.0
1962	13.3	13.9	13.8	14.4
1963	14.7	14.8	14.7	14.9
1964	15.5	15.8	16.0	16.1
1965	16.1	16.4	16.9	16.9
1966	16.6	16.6	16.9	16.9
1967	17.4	17.5	17.3	17.7
1968	17.4	17.5[a]	17.5	17.4
1969	17.6	17.0	16.3	16.0
1970	16.0	16.0	16.2	16.6
1971	16.7	16.6	16.4	16.0
1972	15.6	15.6	15.8	15

Source: United Kingdom, Office of Population Censuses and Surveys. *The Registrar General's Quarterly Return for England and Wales. Quarter ended 31 March, 1973.* London: Her Majesty's Stationery Office, 1973, table IIb, p. 9.

Note: The original birth figures have been adjusted by removing the estimated regular seasonal fluctuations, in order to give a better appreciation of the underlying trend. In assessing the trend, too much significance should not, however, be attached to the figure for one quarter in isolation, because of the considerable random fluctuations that can occur from quarter to quarter, but the general run of figures over a period should be taken into account.

[a]Abortion Act implemented, April 27, 1968.

Concomitant Contraceptive Use

Figure 4-6 shows estimates of 1970 usage of contraception among the approximately 8 million British women aged 15 to 44 then at risk of pregnancy (excluding the pregnant, those trying to get pregnant, subfertile or infertile, or married to a subfertile or infertile partner). By 1965 there was a wide variety of pills on the British market (236). A national survey in 1967-68 showed that 30 percent of women married in the early 1960s had used the pill (127)—the same percentage recorded in 1970 among 350 women interviewed in Hull after five years of marriage (165). However, by 1969 it was reported that only an estimated 16 percent of all married British women were currently using the pill (compared to 22 percent in the United States, as noted), increasing to an estimated 18 percent among *all* women in the fertile age group by the end of

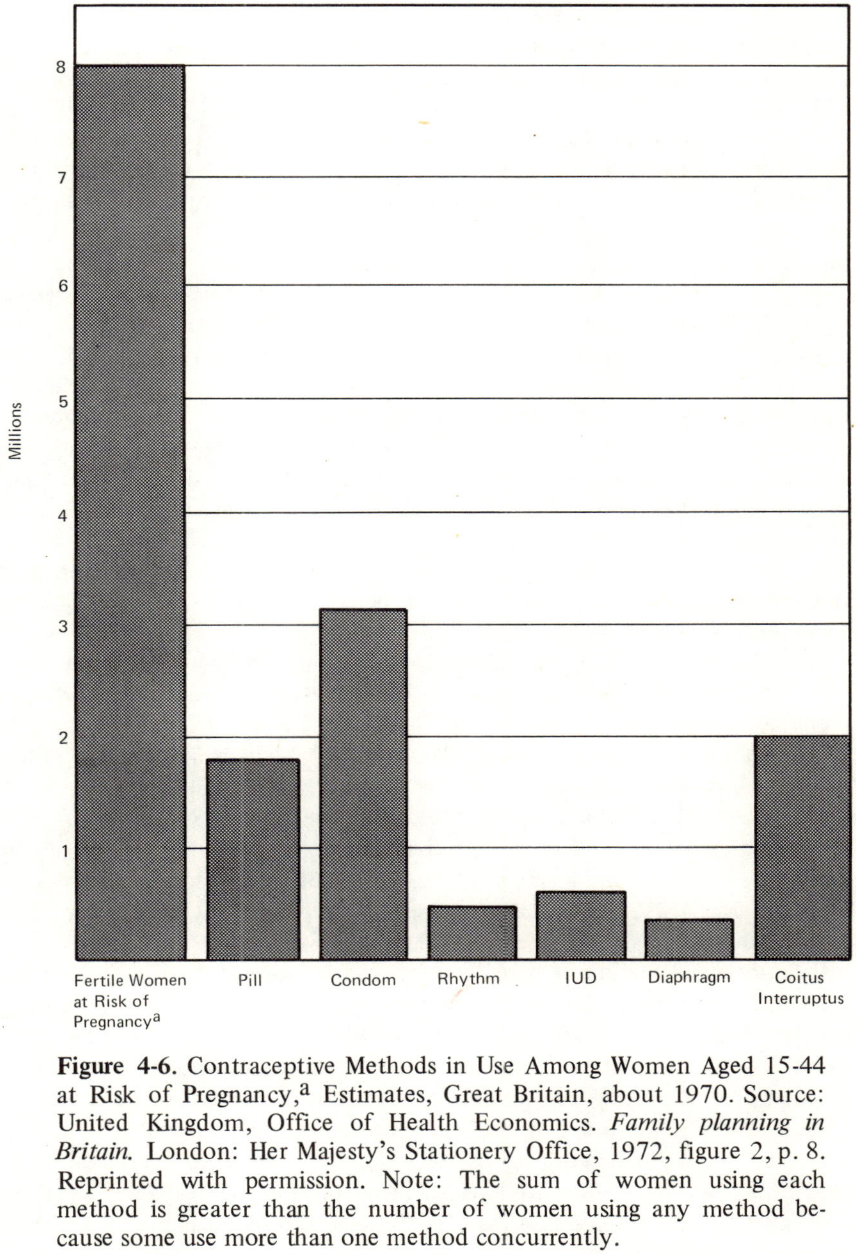

Figure 4-6. Contraceptive Methods in Use Among Women Aged 15-44 at Risk of Pregnancy,[a] Estimates, Great Britain, about 1970. Source: United Kingdom, Office of Health Economics. *Family planning in Britain.* London: Her Majesty's Stationery Office, 1972, figure 2, p. 8. Reprinted with permission. Note: The sum of women using each method is greater than the number of women using any method because some use more than one method concurrently.

[a]Excluding women currently pregnant, trying to get pregnant, subfertile, or infertile, or married to a subfertile or infertile partner.

1971 (236). Condoms remain the most popular contraceptive method, as in Sweden, and coitus interruptus is also used more widely than the pill (267)—by an estimated 2 million couples in 1971, in contrast to 1.8 million women on the pill (236, p. 13).

A 1970 countrywide survey in England and Wales of 2500 women aged 16 to 40 who had ever married or cohabited, and some 1000 single women aged 16 to 35 revealed that in the first group 36 percent of most recent pregnancies were unwanted at the time of conception (22). (This can be compared to the 44 percent of similarly unplanned births occurring from 1966 to 1970, as reported in the U.S. National Fertility Study of 1970.) A 1972 medical report on unplanned pregnancy concluded from this survey and other evidence that although over 90 percent of British married couples are known to have practiced contraception at some time during their married life and contraceptive knowledge has greatly increased among the unmarried, there is a high degree of risk-taking and lack of contraception both within and outside marriage and substantial use of unreliable methods (197). Although not directly queried, it was estimated that among the 1000 single women surveyed in 1970, 33 to 38 percent were sexually experienced, and most of this group were currently active. Only 24 percent of these single women, aged 16 to 35, had ever used contraception: 16 percent condoms, 9 percent the pill, 4 percent coitus interruptus. None had used an IUD.

By 1971, 22 percent of legal aborters in England and Wales were aged under 20 (231, Table 4). Recent information on sexual and contraceptive behavior among teenaged girls, comparable to the 1971 Zelnik-Kantner survey in the United States, is lacking in Britain (166). It is "widely believed" that sexual permissiveness is on the increase among teenagers (89, 197). Two surveys by Kind indicated that the percentage of sexually experienced 18-year-old girls rose from 10-15 in 1963 to 60 in 1968, but the surveyed girls still believed for the most part that it was the man's job to take precautions and many were reckless about the risks (121). Sex education is reported as particularly deficient in boys' schools (197).

Official sanction of family planning came with passage of the Family Planning Act in 1967, in the wake of the abortion act. Numbers of Family Planning Association clinics rose from 613 in 1967 to 1023 in 1971, but in 1970 serviced only 650,000 of the estimated 8 million women at risk of pregnancy, and there is evidence of remaining discrimination in providing services to the unmarried (236). A 1967 survey found widespread reluctance among general practitioners to give unsolicited contraceptive advice (37), and reportedly many still adopt "judgmental attitudes" toward girls receiving the pill (180). Pannell has suggested that "a major accomplishment of the Abortion Act has in fact been the increase in public awareness of the need for effective contraceptive services, for single and married women alike, and for more education in family planning. It has had the effect of putting the final seal of respectability on contraception.

The demand for abortion has also awakened the medical profession to its failure in the past to give proper attention to the prevention of pregnancy" (164, p. 119). From April 1974, family planning services will be provided for the first time within the National Health Service. Patients will be liable only for contraceptive prescription costs (48).

Illegal Abortion Following the 1967 Abortion Act

Annual numbers of deaths attributed to all abortions dropped by half in England and Wales between 1966 and 1972 (53 to 26), suggesting a decline in illegal abortions in the first five years of the new act. However, from 1967 to 1969 deaths following identifiable illegal abortions remained relatively high among black immigrant women in particular (such deaths made up 4.4 percent of deaths from all causes among black women aged 15 to 44, as against 0.3 percent among white women). Also, in London annual figures of hospital emergency admissions for abortion had by 1972 fallen only to 3000, from 4364 in 1967. Potts therefore surmises that illegal abortion has not yet been eradicated (179). He attributes this to residual medical timidity and lack of advertising of abortion facilities (unlike the United States).

Goodhart quotes "guestimates" by presumed authorities which range from 40,000 illegal abortions still in 1970 to "negligible" numbers in 1971 (89). (See Chapter 5 for a discussion of the extent to which legal abortions may merely have replaced illegal abortions in Britain since 1967.)

Singapore

With the inclusion of an "environmental" clause in its 1969 Abortion Act (207, implemented in March 1970), covering a pregnant woman's family and financial circumstances, Singapore became runner-up to the People's Republic of China as the most liberal of non-Western "developing" states to that date. The act was designed not as a substitute for but as a complement to family planning (119), particularly in the case of failed contraception, which had become an embarrassment to family planners faced with women who became pregnant while using officially supplied IUDs (115). Abortions must be authorized by an eleven-member Termination of Pregnancy Authorization Board, who approved 88 percent of 3100 applications received in the first nine months (126). During 1971, the first full year of the act's operation, legal abortions were performed at the rate of 71 per 1000 live births (and at about the same rate in 1972 [120]), compared to 169 in Sweden in that year and 62 in England and Wales in 1969, the first full year under Britain's similar 1967 abortion act (58). An abortion costs about U.S. $1.65 (as does a sterilization—fully authorized for contraceptive purposes also in 1969), compared to U.S. $33 for delivery of a third child and U.S. $82 for a fifth (93).

Age-specific fertility rates fell slightly from 1969 to 1971, but Kee states that "this cannot be solely attributed to legalization of abortion" (119). Since 1957, crude birth rates had declined rapidly in Singapore from 42.4 to 22.1 per 1000 in 1969. The decline from 26.6 in 1966 is claimed as largely attributable to the activities of the official family planning program launched in that year, which by the end of 1970 had reached 64 percent of all married women aged 15 to 44 (118). However, Taeuber points out that "major declines in marital fertility in Singapore between 1957 and 1966 occurred prior to the wide availability of the pill or IUD or legalization of abortion" (223, p. 28), which along with significantly older ages at marriage in these years also helped depress crude birth rates. From 1969 to 1972 numbers of births increased from 44,600 to 49,448, and the crude birth rate increased slightly from 22.1 to an estimated 23.0 (119, 239). This stems from the postwar baby boom. The number of women in the reproductive age group in 1972 was almost double that of 1967 (118).

Kee states that "the impression is" that liberalization of abortion has not diminished contraceptive effort: "There has not been any significant drop in the number of new [family planning] acceptors or in the continuation of those already practicing contraception" (119).

California, Maryland, and Washington State

De Jure Abortion Liberalization

Availability of data makes possible a somewhat detailed comparison of fertility trends in these three U.S. states following abortion law changes with those for the country as a whole in the same period. *California in 1967* and *Maryland in 1968* were among the dozen states which by 1971 had *reformed* their restrictive abortion laws to conform essentially with the Model Penal Code proposed by the American Law Institute in 1955 (8). The key paragraph of this code would permit abortion if a licensed physician "believes there is substantial risk that continuance of the pregnancy would gravely impair the physical or mental health of the mother or that the child would be born with grave physical or mental defects," or if the pregnancy resulted from rape or incest (231). Both states further authorized abortions only in an accredited hospital, following approval by the hospital's review board (32, 135). In *November 1970* the citizens of *Washington state* voted in a *"repeal"* abortion law similar to that of New York, but requiring performance in an approved medical facility, state residency of at least ninety days, no more than seventeen weeks' pregnancy (compared to New York's twenty-four), and consent of a woman's husband if she is living with him, or that of parents or guardian for women aged under 18 (261).

Ensuing Levels of Legal Abortion and Trends in General Fertility Rates

By 1971 the ratio of legal abortions performed in that year on residents to live births six months later (when, on average, the births forestalled by abortion would have occurred) was 331 in California, 215 in Maryland and 286 in Washington, compared to 622 in New York City and 143 in the United States as a whole (231, Table 1). These ratios take into account abortions occurring out of state to residents of the states concerned. This is particularly important in the case of Maryland where, as in most of the states along the northern Atlantic seaboard, large numbers of women traveled to New York to be aborted after July 1970, and to the District of Columbia, where elective abortion became available in 1969 as a result of a court decision in a test case challenging the constitutionality of the District's restrictive abortion law (231). For instance, Maryland residents obtaining legal abortions in D.C. numbered almost 3000 in 1971 and 5561 in 1972 (68).

Figure 4-7 and Table 4-3 portray the trends in general fertility rates (live births per 1000 women aged fifteen to forty-four) in these three states and the United States as a whole from 1966 to 1972, with New York City added for comparison.

In *Maryland*, the general fertility rate had fluctuated slightly above or below that of the United States as a whole from 1960 to 1968 (194), but in 1969, the first year following implementation of the state's abortion reform, this rate fell by 1.5 percent, while the U.S. rate was unchanged from the previous year, and has continued to fall at an accelerating pace, faster than that of the nation at large.

From 1966 to 1970 the general fertility rate for *Washington state* was virtually unchanged, but fell by 13.5 percent during the first year under the new act, more than double the concurrent 6.1 percent drop in the national rate—and the drop in 1972 continued to outstrip that of the nation.

In *California* the possible impact of legalized abortion on fertility trends was delayed. Estimates of illegal abortions prior to 1967, together with other information, suggest that in the first years following passage of the abortion reform law most of the rise in legal abortions represented replacements for illegal abortions (19). However, between 1969 and 1970 numbers of legal abortions quadrupled—15,300 to 65,500—and the state's fertility rate, which had paralleled that of the United States since 1966, dropped dramatically by 11.7 percent in 1971, nearly twice that of the concurrent drop in the U.S. rate.

The general fertility rate in *New York City* had also paralleled that of the

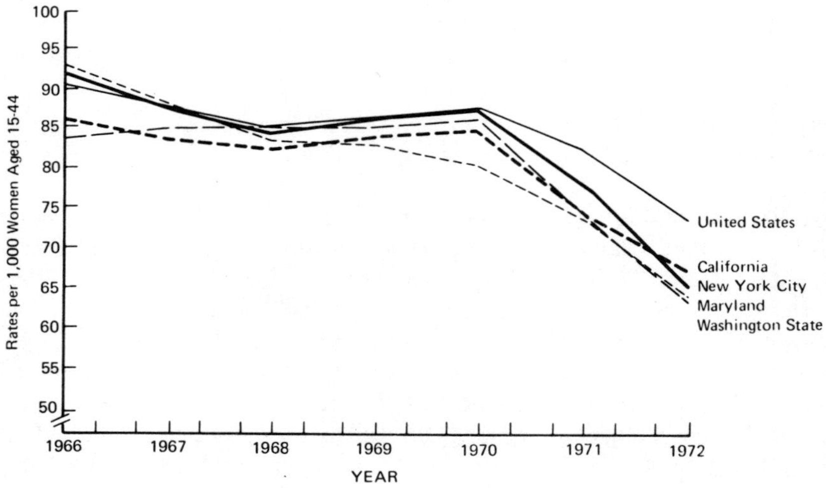

Figure 4-7. General Fertility Rates per 1,000 Women Aged 15-44, United States, California, Maryland, Washington State, and New York City, 1966-72. Source: *California and U.S.:* J. Sklar, and B. Berkov. The effects of legal abortion on legitimate and illegitimate birth rates: the California experience. *Studies in Family Planning*, 1973, 4, table 1, p. 283. *Maryland, 1966-71:* I. Rosenwaike. Therapeutic abortion and fertility in Maryland, 1960-71. Paper presented at Population Association of America Meeting, New Orleans, April 1973, table 1. *New York City:* Computed by C. Tietze, and D.A. Dawson, The Population Council, New York. *Maryland 1972 and Washington State, 1966-72:* Numerators (births) from USDHEW, National Center for Health Statistics. Provisional statistics: Births, deaths, marriages, and divorces: Annual summary for the United States. *Monthly Vital Statistics Report*, issued annually, plus Maryland state records of 1972 out-of-state births occurring to Maryland residents, supplied personally by I. Rosenwaike; denominators (women aged 15-44) 1970 from U.S. Department of Commerce, Bureau of the Census. *1970 Census of Population.* General Population Statistics, PC(1) B22 and B29, table 19; estimates for 1966-69, based on U.S. Department of Commerce, Bureau of the Census. Population estimates and projections. *Current Population Reports*, Series P-25, Nos. 460 and 483, with estimates for intercensal years; estimates for 1971 and 1972, based on U.S. Department of Commerce, Bureau of the Census. Population estimates and projections. *Current Population Reports*, Series P-25, No. 500, May 1973. The latter gives estimates for total population aged 18-44, by state. Sex distribution and ages 15-17 extrapolated from 1970 census data. Note: All births assigned to estimates of women aged 15-44.

Table 4-3
Trends in General Fertility Rates, United States, California, Maryland, Washington State, and New York City, 1966-72

	Live Births per 1,000 Women Aged 15-44									
	Rate					Percent Change in Rate from Previous Year				
Year	U.S.	California	Maryland	Washington State	New York City	U.S.	California	Maryland	Washington State	New York City
1966	91.3	86.3	93.3	84.6*	92.5					
1967	87.6	83.9[a]	87.8	85.5*	87.4	– 4.1	– 2.8	– 5.9	+ 1.1	– 5.5
1968	85.7	82.7	83.9[a]	85.5*	84.4	– 2.2	– 1.4	– 4.9	0.0	– 3.4
1969	86.5	83.9	82.6	85.7*	86.3	+ 0.1	+ 1.5	– 1.5	+ 0.2	+ 2.3
1970	87.6*	84.6	80.8	86.0*[a]	87.3[a]	+ 2.1	+ 0.8	– 2.2	+ 0.4	+ 1.2
1971	82.3*	74.7	73.7	74.4*	76.4	– 6.1	–11.7	– 8.6	–13.5	–12.5
1972	73.4*	67.6	64.7*	64.1*	66.1	–10.8	– 9.5	–13.9	–13.9	–13.5

Sources: Same as for Figure 4-7.

*Provisional

[a]Abortion legalized

nation from 1960 to 1970, but the 1970-71 decline, in the year after the abortion law change, was twice that of the whole country, as in California and Washington. The 1971-72 drop also exceeded that of the national fertility rate.

Of course, the trend in the national fertility rate was undoubtedly also affected by the rise in legal abortions in these years, which by 1972 numbered 586,800 nationwide (231, Table 1), when an estimated 3,256,000 live births occurred (247). However, fertility declines appeared to be accentuated in areas where abortion had been liberalized.

Trends in Out-of-Wedlock Fertility

In California and Washington state, as in New York City (and England and Wales), persuasive evidence that legal abortion was having a significant impact on fertility came from reversals in previous upward trends in out-of-wedlock fertility.

The reversal was particularly sharp in *California*. Between 1970 and 1971, births to unmarried women aged 15 to 44 dropped by 16 percent, from 27 to 22.6 per 1000—a one-year decline equivalent to the five-year increase from 22.5 per 1000 in 1966, when state birth data by legitimacy status were first compiled (19). Three-fourths of legal aborters in the previous year were not currently married.

In *Washington* in the same year—the first year under the new legislation—the proportion of out-of-wedlock births among all births dropped by 7 percent, the first drop in sixteen years and the first drop of more than 1 percent in twenty-two years (184). Women under 20, who accounted for half of out-of-wedlock births, made up 33 percent of legal aborters in that first year.

In *Maryland*, however, the proportion of out-of-wedlock among all births declined among white women following the 1968 abortion law reform, but continued to increase among blacks, although at a slower pace (194). (It should be noted that the proportion of out-of-wedlock among all births [the illegitimacy *ratio*], unlike the number of births per 1000 unmarried women [the illegitimacy *rate*], is affected by trends in legitimate as well as illegitimate fertility and shifts in the proportion of unmarried women. Although the illegitimacy ratio continued to mount among Maryland's black women, a decline might actually have occurred since 1968 in their illegitimacy rate, which is not available.)

Black-White Differentials in Legal Abortion and Fertility, California and Maryland

About 1970, in both California and Maryland the rate of legal abortions per 1000 black women aged 15 to 44 was nearly double that of white women—24.6

among California's black women compared to 13.8 among white women (19), and 19.9 compared to 10.9 in Maryland (194). In the following year, general fertility rates in California declined more for black women than for whites (13.8 as against 11.7 percent), but the reverse was true in Maryland; nonwhite general fertility fell by only 6.1 percent, compared to 9.6 among whites. To account for the lesser decline in nonwhite fertility in Maryland, despite higher abortion rates, Rosenwaike suggests that liberalized abortion may have had a greater impact on fertility trends among whites because nonwhites previously had greater recourse to illegal abortion (194). This possibility is suggested by results of a unique North Carolina survey of 1968 based on the randomized response technique,[a] which produced estimates of one conception in seven among white women resulting in an illegal abortion, compared with one out of three among black women (1). The North Carolina experience may well be applicable to black women in Maryland, with higher levels of legal abortions representing a continuation of the earlier (illegal) pattern, but not so true of black women on the other side of the continent.

Sklar and Berkov remark that what does seem evident in the greater use of legal abortion and continuing higher fertility levels among California black women (as on the East Coast, though fertility differentials are narrowing in California) is that black women make far less use of contraception and thus a greater proportion find themselves with unwanted pregnancies (209). In a study based on a 1969-70 survey of low-income, married or formerly married women in seventeen U.S. cities and comparable data from the 1965 and 1970 National Fertility Studies, Bauman and Udry found the much higher percentages of unwanted births among blacks compared to whites to be associated with lesser use of nonphysician administered contraception (condoms, rhythm, etc.), greater likelihood of no use of contraception, higher failure rates subsequent to adoption of pills or IUDs, and actual lower family-size desires (14). As noted, current use of pills and IUDs (and any contraception) was similar among black and white currently married women interviewed in the 1970 National Fertility Study (266). However, failure rates were much higher among blacks than whites. In the first year of exposure to risk of an unintended pregnancy, 35 percent of black ever-married women compared to 12 percent of similar white women experienced number failures, and timing failures mounted to 39 percent among blacks versus 25 percent among whites (198). Thus, black women in the United States appear to be in Stage 2 of the evolution outlined in Figure 1-1, with falling fertility accomplished chiefly by abortion.

Trends in Marriages, and Births and Abortions Among Teenagers

That legal abortion is now being used to terminate substantial numbers of pregnancies among unmarried women that formerly would have led to forced mar-

---

[a]For an explanation of this technique for collecting survey information on sensitive topics see Tietze and Dawson (231, p. 4).

riages is suggested by a reversal of previous upward trends in numbers of marriages and the marriage rate in Washington and Maryland since abortion law changes (as in the District of Columbia since 1969, and in New York in the first year following the 1970 abortion change), and in California in 1971 following the large 1969-70 upsurge in legal abortions. This occurred despite a continuing swell of postwar baby-boomers entering the most marriageable ages, 18 to 24, and in contrast to an unbroken upward trend in marriages nationally since 1958 (247). In Washington state the proportion of teenaged marriages decreased significantly from 1970 to 1972 (184).

Also in California, in both 1971 and 1972, there was a sharp drop in the previously rising numbers of births among married teenagers—up to two-fifths of which can be assumed to be premaritally conceived (248). Together with the concurrent sharp rise in legal abortion rates among unwed teenagers, this suggests to Sklar and Berkov that the increased availability of legal abortion has significantly reduced the rate of "shotgun" marriages among California's teenagers (209).

Subsequent Developments in California

After the dramatic fertility drops of 1971, the picture changed in California in 1972. Marital fertility rates declined no faster than in 1971 (about 10 percent in both years), while the rate of out-of-wedlock fertility declined by only 2.7 percent, compared to the 16 percent drop of the previous year. Meanwhile, the climb in abortion rates slowed to 30.4 percent, in contrast to the previous year's 146 percent, and in the following twelve months is estimated to have leveled off almost completely (209, p. 283, fn). Sklar and Berkov conclude that if California's experience is used as a criterion, legal abortion, in the United States at any rate, may continue to have future importance in reducing fertility both in and out of wedlock, but this could dwindle after an initial sharp impact. In 1972, California's legitimate births numbered 59,650 fewer than might have been expected on the basis of 1966-70 trends; substantially more than the 30,500 legal abortions obtained by married women in the period affecting those births. Thus it is clear that large numbers of married women in California are limiting their fertility by means other than legal abortion. However, in the same period, legal abortions among California's unmarried women amounted to 82,600—far outstripping the almost 12,000 additional out-of-wedlock births that might have been expected in 1972 had 1966-70 rising trends continued. Thus, legal abortion is clearly "keeping a lid on" what otherwise would be a continuing rise in the rate of out-of-wedlock childbearing (209).

5 Fertility Impact of Illegal but Widely Practiced Abortion

A combination of criminal abortions and contraception in restrictive countries that are economically and technologically advanced, and in those that are starting to develop or are semi-developed also lowers birth rates, but not so rapidly. (33, pp. 291-92)

Western Industrialized Countries with Restrictive Abortion

The birth rates of most Western industrialized countries share a common pattern. At the time of the Depression, between the two World Wars, the birth rates of industrialized nations fell to a low level—often as low as, or lower than, that current today. Commonly the age of marriage was somewhat higher, but this factor alone does not account for the low fertility and it must be assumed that the total numbers of births averted (by combined use of contraception and abortion) was of the same order of magnitude in the later 1920s and 1930s as it is today. However, there can be no doubt that the availability, use and effectiveness of contraceptive methods, as well as the resort to sterilization, have all increased considerably over the past forty years. Therefore, abortion was probably a more important factor in fertility control than at the present time. (182, Chapter 11)

United States before 1967

Birth Rates, Contraceptive Use, and Abortion "Guestimates" During the 1930s. During the 1930s U.S. birth rates dropped to the lowest level recorded to that time, an average of just over 17 per 1000 population—depths to which birth rates did not again fall until 1968 (240). Campbell has shown that the decline in fertility was actually more rapid during the 1920s than during the Depression years of the early 1930s, and culminated in the record low fertility of the women born from 1906 to 1910. These women bore on average just 2.3 children, and 22 percent remained childless (35).

A 1938-39 study of the Market Research Corporation and a 1941 Indianapolis survey of white Protestant married women revealed that 30 to 44 percent of contracepting couples relied solely on douching, with a much lower percentage reporting condom or diaphragm use. Coitus interruptus was infrequently mentioned in either of these studies. Campbell remarks:

In view of what we now know about the ineffectiveness of douching and about the irregularity with which later cohorts have used the condom and diaphragm, it hardly seems possible for the cohorts of 1906-1910, as well as other cohorts in their reproductive years during the 1920s and 1930s, to have achieved such low fertility with the methods then in common use. It seems probable that there was widespread resort to illegal abortion in these decades. (35, pp. 107-108)

The most-cited authority on abortions during the 1930s estimated an annual ratio of 1 abortion per approximately 2.5 live births in cities and 1 per 5 live births in rural areas, yielding a national total of 681,000 abortions. Some 60 to 65 percent were assumed to be illegal (F.J. Taussig, *Abortion: Spontaneous and Induced*, St. Louis, 1936, quoted in 33, p. 133).

Post-World War II Trends in Birth Rates, Contraceptive Use, and Abortion. Figure 2-9 indicates that following World War II U.S. birth rates fluctuated at a steady level until 1957–about 25 per 1000, well above the prewar level of about 17 per 1000–and thereafter declined steadily, although at a much lesser pace than in Japan during the decade following its 1948 abortion liberalization. The U.S. birth rate fell to 17.8 in 1967, 15.6 in 1971 (59 percent of the 1947 rate of 26.6; see Figure 2-9), and for the first half of 1973 reached the record low level of 14.8 per 1000 (249). Among developed countries, only Canada, Australia, and New Zealand rivaled the United States in the height and length of its postwar baby boom (35). Nevertheless, during this period contraceptive use was rising, together with estimates of resort to illegal abortion (*and* women's educational attainment and employment [35]; see also Appendix table).

National surveys of white Catholic and Protestant currently married women conducted in 1955, 1960, and 1965 reported percentages of those who had used or expected to use contraception at 79, 87, and 90 respectively. Confined to fecund couples, the percentages rise to 91, 96, and 97 (Growth of American Families 1955 and 1960, and National Fertility Study 1965, cited in 199, Table V-8). Among white women who had ever used contraception, the preferred methods reported in 1960 were condoms (50 percent), diaphragm (38 percent) and rhythm (35 percent). By 1965, among contraceptors, 33 percent of white married women and 29 percent of nonwhite married women had used the pill. Coitus interruptus–never a popular method in the United States–had been used by only 15-20 percent of both races, about the same level reported in the two earlier surveys (199, Table V-17). However, in 1965 at least one-third of fecund couples still used no contraception or relied on methods of "doubtful effectiveness" (110), and three-fifths reported having had births that were not wanted at all or wanted later (compared to the 44 percent of such unplanned births occurring from 1966 to 1970, as reported in the National Fertility Study of 1970).

In the mid-1950s, national estimates of induced abortions ranged from 200,000 to 1,200,000 (Arden House Conference on Abortions, cited in 31, p.

180). For the period just prior to adoption of moderate abortion laws by some states beginning in 1967, Tietze states that "constant repetition has led to the wide acceptance of a round figure of 1 million induced abortions per year [of which only an estimated 8000 were legal], corresponding to an abortion rate of 5 per 1000 population and an abortion ratio of almost 30 per 100 live births" (227). These estimated abortion rates and ratios are almost double those based on legal abortions performed on residents in England and Wales in 1972, five years after abortion legalization—2.2 per 1000 population and 15.0 per 100 live births, respectively. They are also nearly double the figures based on the 586,800 legal abortions recorded for 1972 in the United States as a whole—2.8 per 1000 population and 18.0 per 100 live births (58).

Age at Marriage. The average age of U.S. women upon their first marriage has varied less in these decades than is commonly supposed. Goode cites 21 as the average in 1920, 1930, and 1940. This dropped to just over age 20 in 1959 and in March 1973 was again 21 (87; 246, Table D). Thus, age at marriage could have had little impact on the trend in crude birth rates in this time period.

Great Britain before 1967

Contraception, Abortion "Guestimates," Birth Rates, and Age at Marriage. Historical evidence is available to show that the decline in British birth rates starting in 1877—the year of the Bradlaugh-Besant trial—was associated with both adoption of contraception *and* increased resort to abortion (167). (Widespread publicity surrounding this lengthy trial of two well-known public figures who had deliberately reprinted and sold a U.S. contraceptive pamphlet spread the gospel of family limitation and created a demand for contraception among late Victorians, who for complex social and psychological reasons were especially ready at that time to receive such a message [168].) In the 1930s, birth rates in England and Wales averaged 14-15 per 1000, and about 18 per 1000 in Scotland. In England and Wales the rate dropped down to this level again in 1954 and 1955 (15.2, 15.0), rose to 18.8 in 1964, and has since declined to 14.7 in 1972. After the 1930s the Scottish birth rate remained steady at a slightly higher level—18 to 20 per 1000—until 1969, when it dropped slightly to 17.4, declining further to 16.6 in 1971, a bit below the level of the 1930s (239, 240).

For both English and Scottish women the average age at marriage was somewhat over 25 during the 1930s, and thus may have been a factor in the relatively low crude birth rates of that decade. By 1951 the average had dropped to 21.3 in England and Wales and 22.6 in Scotland (21, Table 11-1). However, the English crude birth rate dipped in the next few years, while that of Scotland remained steady. The English average age at marriage rose slightly to 21.8 in 1960 (69, Table 1), but the birth rate also mounted slightly in the early 1960s

(Figure 4-4). Thus it would appear that age at marriage, at least in recent decades, has been of no significance in British birth rate trends.

A 1946 national survey of mostly lower-income married women indicated a rising use of contraception during the first third of the twentieth century, from 15 percent among women married before 1910 to 66 percent among those married in the latter half of the 1930s (133). Among couples married in the 1950s, 74 percent reported use of contraception at some time, with 45 percent starting contraception at marriage, compared to only 36 percent of those first married in the 1930s (Population Investigation Committee Survey 1959, quoted in 168, p. 25). Coitus interruptus was by far the single most common method until its gradual replacement by condoms and other appliances among couples married in the 1940s and later (178).

Meanwhile, an Interdepartmental Committee on Abortion reported in 1939 that they had found a "widespread conviction [among] persons competent to form a judgement" (police, doctors and the like) that there had been a marked increase in the frequency of abortion (167, p. 6). For the 1930s the committee estimated a national total of 110,000-150,000 abortions annually, 40 percent illegal. At this time there were approximately 600,000 births annually (182). In the Camberwell district of London, annual abortion admissions to St. Giles Hospital rose from 147 in 1924 to 293 in 1934. Over the same period the birth rate in the area fell from 18.2 to 13.2 per 1000 (T. Parish, *British Journal of Obstetrics and Gynaecology*, 1935, quoted in 167).

Estimates of 1960-67 Levels of Abortion, and Extent to Which Post-1967 Legal Abortions Represent Replacements of Illegal Abortion. During the 1960s, before the new abortion act came into force at the end of April 1968, legal abortions performed in English and Welsh National Health Service hospitals and privately are estimated to have risen from 14,300 in 1960 to 27,200 in 1967 (67). In addition to this, the most widely quoted "guestimate" of annual illegal abortions–for England and Wales and Scotland combined–was 100,000 (111). Basing his analysis on data from maternal deaths, hospital admissions, a 1966 National Opinion Poll, and evidence from Aberdeen in Scotland, where a liberal abortion policy was practiced prior to the act, Goodhart argues that no more than 10,000 to 20,000 illegal abortions occurred annually before the law was changed (88, 89). James has used the same data to arrive at a total of 60,000 and upward (111).

If the latter is taken as the more plausible approximation of pre-1968 illegal abortions and added to the some 27,000 legal abortions of 1967, it suggests that the great majority of the 116,200 legal abortions performed on British residents (England, Wales, and Scotland) in 1972–nearly five years after implementation of the 1967 Abortion Act–would have taken place with no change in the law. In that case the act's impact on fertility trends is dubious and it would seem fair to assume, as suggested in the quote heading this section, that the weight has indeed shifted from abortion to contraception in the fertility control that has dropped recent British birth rates down to or below the low levels of the 1930s. On the other hand, Goodhart's far lower assumption of no more than 20,000 illegal abortions annually prior to the act, added to some 27,000 legal abortions, would indicate that the far higher and rising numbers of current legal abortions largely represent an entirely new demand, with significant implications for current and future fertility trends in Britain.

It does seem clear that the abortion act probably resulted in more access to abortion among the young and unmarried than was formerly possible. British public attitudes have until recently militated against the seeking and receiving of contraceptive advice among this group (167), and in the preact era criminal abortionists were less eager to deal with such women, as they tended to seek help late in pregnancy (67). Peel and Potts suggest that in the currently changing pattern of British premarital sexual behavior, the young unmarried appear to be reenacting the probable pre-World War I (and later) experience of the married, with poor contraceptive use and frequent recourse to abortion (167). Thus they appear to be in Stage 2 of the abortion-contraception-fertility model portrayed in Figure 1-1, while British married women have moved on to the final stage of low birth rates, achieved mainly by contraception, with abortion resorted to only in the case of contraceptive failure (or perhaps negligence, if the contraceptive habits of the married in Britain are careless to the extent indicated in the United States by the 1970 National Fertility Study mentioned above). By 1971-72, about a fifth of British legal aborters were teenagers and well over half were unmarried (231, Tables 4 and 9). As noted, legalized abortion does seem to have been effective in braking what otherwise would be a continuing rise in out-of-wedlock and premaritally-conceived births.

Western and Southern Europe

Abortion Levels, Contraceptive Use, and Fertility Trends. In Western and Southern Europe legal abortion is normally still restricted technically to pregnancies that threaten a woman's life, and until recently has been regarded with general hostility (100,179). (By late 1973 the parliaments of Austria and France were debating new bills to ease currently punitive abortion laws, and law reform was an impassioned public issue in at least Switzerland, Italy, and The Netherlands.) However, many of these countries have a long history of low birth rates and "it is generally assumed that [they] have for many years relied upon induced abortion to prevent births—as a supplement in the past to abstinence, withdrawal and crude forms of contraception" (146, Chapter 11). Recent data suggest that the gradually declining birth rates in most of these countries (Figure 2-8)—after a relative rise in at least Italy, Switzerland, and France to the mid-1960s—are also largely effected by a continuing combination of traditional contraceptive methods and illegal (though now rarely penalized [100]) abortion. For about 1967, Table 5-1 shows the relationship between availability of contraception requiring supplies in Western and Southern European countries, the estimated ratio of illegal abortions to births as gleaned from the literature by Hubinont et al. (100), and crude birth rates. The only birth rates exceeding 20 per 1000 are found in Portugal, Spain, and Ireland, with apparently relatively little illegal abortion (though the authors consider the Spanish abortion estimates "suspiciously low") and contraception officially unavailable. In the five countries with illegal abortions estimated at one or more per live birth–Austria, Belgium, Italy, the Federal Republic of Germany, and France–contraception was officially still unsanctioned or only recently available in 1967, and birth rates exceeded 18 per 1000 only in Italy.

In 1969, despite the recent availability of contraceptive supplies, coitus interruptus and rhythm were still the most commonly used methods in Italy, Belgium, and France, according to a five-country family planning study (106). Only in Western Germany had pill usage reached high levels (34 percent of a

Table 5-1
Estimated Ratio of Illegal Abortions to Births in Western and Southern Europe in Relation to the Availability of Contraception about 1967 and Birth Rates for 1967

Availability of Contraception	Country	Estimated Illegal Abortions/Births	Live Births per 1,000 Population
		(range)	
Not available	Austria	1:1 - 3:1	17.4
	Greece	1:3	18.7
	Portugal	1:10	21.5
	Spain	1:47	21.0
	Ireland	"very low"	21.1
Recently available	Belgium	1:3 - 1:1	15.3
	Italy	1:6 - 1:1	18.1
	France	1:3 - 1.5:1	17.0
	Federal Republic of Germany	1:1	14.8
Freely available	Great Britain	1:10- 1:4	17.5
	Netherlands	1:10- 1:3	18.9
	Switzerland	1:10- 1:5	17.7

Sources: P.O. Hubinont, T. Brat, J. Polderman, and R. Ramdoyal, Abortion in Western Europe. In R.E. Hall (ed.), *Abortion in a changing world.* Vol. 1. New York: Columbia University Press, 1970, table 12, p. 336, based on estimates cited in the literature.

1967 crude birth rates–United Nations, Statistical Office. *Demographic yearbook 1969.* New York: Author, 1970, table 12, p. 256.

sample of 830 women), which Potts comments "may have marginal effect in cutting the induced abortion rate" (179). Hervet reported of *France* in 1970 that surveys indicated pill use by only 6 percent of married women (although it was 16 percent among the 819 married French women in the 1969 five-country survey just mentioned). Fifty percent of contracepting women still used coitus interruptus and 20 percent condoms, with abortion apparently still widely relied upon as a backstop. Moreover, though still illegal, abortion procedures are becoming increasingly safe (and unpunished) in France (96).

In *Greece*, Valaoras states that "induced abortion represents the most important factor" (253) in the decline of total fertility rates per woman from 3.7 in the 1930s to 2.3 in the 1960s (179). (The total fertility rate per woman is an estimate of the number of children a woman would bear if she went through her reproductive years exposed to the fertility rates by age prevailing at a particular time, and did not die before the end of this period. A total fertility rate of 2.3 means that parents are just slightly more than replacing themselves.) A 1966 national survey of 0.5 percent of fertile couples in the country disclosed 1 abortion to 5 live births in villages and 1 to 1 in Athens. Forty percent of surveyed women used abortion as the preferred method of family limitation, in contrast to roughly a third using coitus interruptus and another third using other traditional methods or no contraception (253).

In *Italy* in the mid-1960s birth rates varied from 24.1 per 1000 in Calabria in the south to 13.4 per 1000 in the Piedmont, suggesting that northern Italy shares the fertility regulation practices of its near neighbors in France, Germany, Switzerland, and Northern Yugoslavia (where abortion is legal). The ratio of hospital admissions for septic abortions to deliveries can run as high as one to three in some Northern Italian urban areas (179).

In Switzerland and The Netherlands, abortion under acceptable medical conditions is increasingly available in large urban centers from doctors who either interpret restrictive legal indications liberally or apparently flout the law with impunity.

In *Switzerland* in 1966, 110,700 live births were registered in comparison with 21,800 *legal* abortions, including those obtained by nonresidents–90 percent performed in the five largest cities–and possibly another 50,000 illegal abortions occurred (211).

In *The Netherlands*, an abrupt change in attitudes toward abortion since 1967 has led to a sharp increase in estimated annual numbers of abortions obtained by Dutch women from doctors, from well under 20,000 in the early 1960s to well over 30,000 in 1970-71, performed in hospitals, the nine non-profit-making clinics operating by early 1972, and in Britain (800 in 1970 and 850 in 1971 [238]). A study by Treffers reveals that this increase in abortions is associated with an unexpected drop in crude birth rates and general fertility rates from 18.9 and 145.6 respectively in 1969 to 17.2 and 129.9 in 1971 (233). (The birth rate fell further, to 16.1, in 1972 [239] .) Unlike the earlier fertility drop of

1965 and 1966 following introduction of the pill to The Netherlands in 1964, Treffers feels these drops cannot be explained by a further sudden increase in adoption of modern contraception (although Fabery estimates from sales figures that by 1971 22 percent of Dutch women of childbearing age were on the pill, and notes that condoms became widely available through slot machines in 1970 [71]). Use of IUDs and sterilization has increased gradually in recent years, but these methods can account for little or none of the drop of 5000 in first births between 1969 and 1971, which accounts for 25 percent of the decline in these two years. Equally unlikely is that IUDs and sterilization were responsible for the sudden reversal in 1969 of a decade-long rise in absolute numbers and ratios of out-of-wedlock births, or a 1971 drop in premaritally conceived births (71).

That medically obtained abortions are not simply replacing illegal abortions is concluded from the large excess of current abortions over estimates of illegal abortions in the early 1960s, and the fact that studies show that in 1971 unmarried women comprised 40 percent of abortees in several abortion clinics and one large hospital, compared to 19 percent among patients with abortion complications in the same hospital in 1962-64. Treffers attributes the increased demand for abortion in The Netherlands to the introduction of new efficient contraceptive methods, which, as "verified in many studies," puts the possibility of pregnancy planning suddenly within reach of a large group of the population to whom an unwanted or untimely pregnancy now becomes unacceptable (233).

Abortion Interaction Between Western European Countries. Increasing numbers of Western European women "with money or initiative" are now seeking abortions in countries with more liberal attitudes or policies, especially in some cantons of Switzerland (Geneva in particular), The Netherlands, and Britain—a process that Potts points out has in the past "always been a stimulus to national reform" (179). For instance, between October 1971 and February 1972 an estimated 1500 foreign women obtained abortions from doctors in The Hague (233). By 1971 the ratio of abortions performed in Britain on women coming from the Continent, to live births in the countries concerned, was approaching half the 1969 ratio for British women immediately after the 1967 Abortion Act came into force (179, Table 9).

Socioeconomic Development, Infant Mortality, and Desired Family Size. Socioeconomic development, already at a relatively high level, continued at an accelerating speed in the 1950s and 1960s in Western Europe generally (see Appendix table), even spreading to the fringes—Portugal, Spain, Ireland, and Southern Italy. Combined with levels of infant mortality that were already low in most cases and urban housing shortages in some countries, it is to be expected that these conditions enhanced generally long-time low family-size ideals in this region and the continuing necessity for strict fertility control, by whatever means possible. It should be noted, however, that average ideal family sizes reported during the 1960s range from 2.5 to 3 in Western Europe (including Great Britain), while in Eastern Europe the average was scarcely above 2 (Appendix table).

Developing Countries with Restrictive Abortion

When developing societies are highly motivated to accelerate their transition from high to low fertility, induced abortion becomes such a popular method of fertility control that it becomes a kind of epidemic. (160, p. 481)

Republic of Korea and Taiwan

In the Republic of Korea and Taiwan, despite restrictive abortion laws, the incidence of abortion rose along with increasing use of modern contraception during the 1960s, and is acknowledged as having played a significant role in recent dramatic fertility declines. Nationwide family-planning programs were launched in Korea in 1962 and Taiwan in 1964, at a time of social change, rapid population growth (partially due to rapid in-migration following the Korean War and the Chinese Civil War), rising ages at marriage and educational level, and increasing pressure to control family size, especially in overcrowded urban areas—despite some common cultural aspects favoring fertility, particularly a strong desire for sons (182, Chapter 11). Primary emphasis has been on the IUD, with pills introduced in Taiwan in 1967 and in Korea in 1968.

Status and Availability of Abortion. Abortion for any reason is still illegal in Taiwan, although reform is under consideration (45), and was technically permitted in Korea only for strict medical reasons until January 1973. It is now also legal in cases of rape, incest, and risk of a deformed fetus (124). In principle, abortion is widely disapproved. In 1970, disapproval was expressed by 65 percent of Taiwanese women approached in an islandwide family-planning study (216) and 88 percent of women surveyed in Seoul, Korea (98), although by only 54 percent of women in Korea's national Fertility-Abortion Survey of the following year (144). In practice, abortions are widely available privately from physicians, who performed virtually all abortions in Seoul in 1970 (98) and 80 percent in Taiwan in 1969, with the remainder being done by midwives at maternity homes (44). Costs are low, ranging from U.S. $7.50 to U.S. $9.00 in Seoul between 1964 and 1970, and about U.S. $4.50 in Korean rural areas in 1965 (98).

Birth Rate Declines and Proportions Attributable to Contraception and Abortion. Birth rates were already declining in both countries before 1960, but the drops from 1960 to 1970 were dramatic (although with a slowdown after 1968). Korea's birth rate dropped 28-32 percent from an estimated 42.9 to 29-31 per 1000 population, and the drop was 31 percent in Taiwan—from 39.5 to 27.2 per 1000 (Table 5-2). (Taiwan's birth rate fell further to 24.2 by 1972 [270], while according to some authorities Korea's birth rate has stabilized at about 31 [39]. However, a late 1973 nationwide sample survey indicates a crude birth rate of 28.0 for 1971-73 [263].) In both cases, about 40 percent of the ten-year decline can be attributed to changes in the age-sex structure of the population and rising ages at marriage (42, 43, 81). Of the remaining 60 percent, in *Korea*, one report attributes a little more than half to contraception and a little less than half to abortion (B.-M. Lee, quoted in 264), while another attributes 63 percent to contraception and the remainder to illegal abortion (Smith and Watson, 1972, quoted in 182, Chapter 11). Based on data gathered in the 1971 national Fertility-Abortion Survey of 6300 women, Hong calculates that without induced abortion Korea's 1970 crude birth rate would have been 33 rather than an estimated 29 per 1000 population (99). For *Taiwan*, theoretical considerations suggest that use of contraception supplied through the national program would account for an estimated decline in the birth rate from the known level of 36.6 in 1963 to a theoretical level of 32.0 in 1969. The 1969 level was in fact 27.7. Potts, Diggory, and Peel point out that the difference is due to the effects of commercial distribution of contraceptives and of illegal abortion. "Unfortunately, no effort has been made to partition these two factors" (182, Chapter 11). However, information on induced abortion rates is available in Taiwan as for Korea. (Kee and Lee state that in Taiwan in recent years up to half of oral pills used have come from commercial sources [120], but in 1970 only an estimated 3.3 percent of women of childbearing ages were currently using the pill [Table 5-2].)

Contraceptive Use in the 1960s. In *Korea* less than 5 percent of eligible couples were practicing family limitation prior to 1962 (91). As seen in Table 5-2, nationwide surveys indicated that the percentage of married women of childbearing age *currently* practicing contraception mounted from 9 in 1964 to 25 in 1971, when 44 percent reported having used contraception at some time. By 1971, 25 percent had used the pill at some time and another 25 percent the IUD, but *current* use was only 7 percent for each method, with another 4 percent of couples sterilized. Current contraceptive use percentages have been higher in *Taiwan*: reportedly 34 percent in 1967, rising to 44 percent by early 1970, with approximately 20 percent using IUDs, but only a low 3.3 percent regular users of pills (132).

IUD and pill discontinuation rates are high in both countries. In *Korea* 1969 national data show continuation rates after one year of only 30 percent for pills and 58 percent for IUDs (264). Similar data for *Taiwan* for the period 1965-68 put the percentages at 25 for pills and 60 for IUDs (217, Tables 1 and 12).

However, followup surveys also disclose that in Korea 40 percent of pregnancies occurring up to three years following insertion of an IUD were deliberately aborted (196) and in Taiwan "about three-quarters" of all such pregnancies are terminated by induced abortion (269, p. 64). Many of these pregnancies occurred with the IUD still in place, and the proportions terminated by abortion in these circumstances are far higher than for pregnancies occurring otherwise. Ross et al. point out that, thus, "abortion has been used increasingly to compensate for contraceptive failure rather than as a primary method to limit births; hence it accounts for less substitution effect and more net births prevented" (195, p. 37).

Prevalence of Abortion in the 1960s. In *Korea*, national data indicate that the percentage of married women aged 15 to 49 having resorted to abortion more than quadrupled between 1964 and 1971–6 to 26 percent (Table 5-2). Watson observes that, thus, in 1971, after a decade of organized family planning, more Korean women reported having had at least one abortion (26 percent) than ever having used an IUD or the pill (25 percent each; Table 5-2). Among women aged 15 to 54 the percentages reported in 1971 were 24 percent abortion, 19 percent IUD, and 18 percent the pill (262).

In *Taiwan*, similar data document a rise from 9.5 percent in 1965 to 13.8 percent in 1970 (Table 5-2). Direct surveys in Taiwan at least probably "grossly underestimate the true incidence of abortion," according to Chow (44, p. 252). A randomized response test administered in April 1970 to a sample of some 1000 women in a county of northern Taiwan indicated that about 28.2 percent of this group had had induced abortions (similar to the Korean level), compared to 12.7 percent admitted among a comparable group in response to direct questioning (45). (This investigation formed part of the "Epidemiological Study on the Outcome of Pregnancy," data from which are to be used together with information from previous family-planning surveys and a current survey of public leaders and medical professionals in a study by L.P. Chow and colleagues of the Department of Population Dynamics, The Johns Hopkins University, Baltimore, on "The Impact of Reform of Abortion Laws in Taiwan," which seeks to gauge the potential impact of abortion law reform on fertility trends, health of the people and health and medical care systems, and contraceptive acceptance and continuation. Preliminary results expected in 1974 [46].)

Rural-Urban Differentials in Abortion and Fertility. In both countries, "as in all similar studies elsewhere" (44), levels of abortion are higher in urban than in rural areas. (The incidence of abortion was higher in urban areas–especially in larger cities–than in rural areas in all of the eight countries for which Tietze and Dawson report such data: Czechoslovakia, England and Wales, Greece, Hungary, Japan, Korea, Sweden, and Turkey [231, Tables 1-3].) In *Korea* in 1965 and 1971, 23 and 34 percent of urban women (40 percent in Seoul in 1971)

Table 5-2
Birth Rates, and Prevalence of Abortion and Contraception Among Married Women of Childbearing Age,[a] Republic of Korea and Taiwan, 1960-71

	Births per 1,000 Population		% Married Women Having Had at Least One Abortion		% Married Women Currently Using						% Married Women Who Have Ever Used					
					Contraception		Pill		IUD		Contraception		Pill		IUD	
	Year	Rate	Year	%	Year	%	Year	%	Year	%	Year	%	Year	%	Year	%
Republic of Korea	1960	42.9														
			1965	11	1964	9					1964	12				
			1967	20	1967	20	1966	1	1966	9	1967	28				
	1970	29.0-31.0	1971	26	1971	25	1971	7	1971	7	1971	44	1971	25	1971	25
Percent decline in birth rate		28 - 32														
Taiwan	1960	39.7														
			1965	9.5	1965	22.8					1965	28.1			1965	10.2
			1967	12.3	1968	33.5					1965	41.1				
	1970	27.2	1970	13.8	1970	44.1	1970	3.3	1970	20	1970	55.5	1970	11	1970	33.9
Percent decline in birth rate		31.0														

[a]The age range of women included varied among the surveys from which these data are derived, but generally covered at least women currently aged 20-49. All women surveyed were currently or had been married.

Sources:

Republic of Korea: K.S. Chang, G.C. Worth, W.B. Watson, and P.H. Michael, Korea (South). *Studies in Family Planning*, 1973, 4, 107-11; L.-J. Cho. Economic and demographic influences on the family in Korea. In National Institutes of Health, Fogarty International Center, *The family in transition: A round table conference*, Bethesda, Maryland, November 1969. Washington: U.S. Government Printing Office, Fogarty International Center Proceedings No. 3, 1971, pp. 139-54; L.-J. Cho. The demographic situation in the Republic of Korea. Paper presented at the Population Association of America Meeting, New Orleans, Louisiana, April 1973; H.-S. Moon, S.-H. Han, and S. Choi. *Fertility and family planning: An interim report on 1971 fertility-abortion survey.* Seoul: Korean Institute for Family Planning, 1973, tables III-20, III-36, III-37, III-38, III-40.

Taiwan: L.P. Chow. Measurement of the incidence of abortion: Preliminary results from a study in Taiwan. Paper presented at the International Union for the Scientific Study of Population, Workshop on Abortion, University of North Carolina, Chapel Hill, March 1973, table 2; R. Freedman, L.C. Coombs, and M.-C. Chang. Trends in family-size preferences and practice of family planning: Taiwan, 1965-1970. *Studies in Family Planning*, 1972, 3, table 13, and p. 291; T.Y. Lee. Taiwan. *Studies in Family Planning*, 1972, 3, 145-50; J.A. Ross, A. Germain, J.E. Forrest, and J. van Ginneken. Findings from family planning research. *Reports on Population/Family Planning*, October 1972, No. 12, table 2, and p. 8.

reported having had abortions compared to 5 and 19 percent in rural areas (144, Table 111-20). The family-planning program has been aimed chiefly at rural areas, and abortion has become common there only quite recently (269). In *Taiwan* according to a 1966-67 Vital Registration Survey, the number of abortions per 1000 live births was 134 in large cities, 94 in towns, and 60 in rural areas (44, p. 253).

In *Korea* by 1971, according to that year's Fertility-Abortion Survey, crude birth rates were the same in urban and rural areas (28.9 and 28.8 respectively), but Watson points out that a deficit of women aged 20 to 34 in rural areas–in contrast to a surplus at these ages in urban areas, particularly in Seoul (due to rural-urban migration)–probably holds down rural rates and pushes up urban rates (262). Women surveyed in Seoul reported an average of 3.2 live births and 0.95 induced abortions up to 1971, while the average among rural women was 4.6 live births and only a third as many induced abortions–0.32 (92, Table III-4). By 1969 in *Taiwan* the urban total fertility rate was still substantially lower than the rural rate–3.2 births per woman in Taipei, compared to 4.1 in towns and 4.6 in rural areas (81, Table 6).

Social Class Differentials in Abortion and Fertility. In both Korea and Taiwan, studies of the late 1960s and early 1970s generally still reveal the highest levels of abortion and lowest fertility among the best educated and most economically advanced women. In *Taiwan*, about 1966-67, the proportion of women who had experienced at least one abortion increased from 9 percent for those with no formal education, to 14 percent for those with a primary-school education, to 18 percent for women having completed junior high school (44, Table 4), while the total fertility rate declined from 5.5 among the illiterate to 2.6 per woman among senior school graduates (81, p. 151). However, two surveys of 1964 and 1970 in the large Sungdong-Gu district of Seoul suggest a "democratization of abortion" process (98), as seen also in Santiago, Chile (below), and illustrated in Figure 1-1. Although in 1970 abortion was still more prevalent among this area's better-educated women (as in a rural survey of 1965 in Korea [97]), the greatest increase in abortion in these years, both relative and absolute, had occurred among the least educated (Figure 5-1). In Seoul in general, when divided roughly by socioeconomic level of the different areas, the 1971 Fertility-Abortion Survey indicated crude births rates among lower class districts still nearly double those of the highest level (33 compared to 17 per 1000 population), with 31 percent of women in lower-class areas ever having had an abortion compared to 44 percent in the most economically advanced areas, but nearly equal levels of pill and IUD use (Table 5-3).

Han's analysis of countrywide abortion data from this 1971 Korean survey also shows that among younger married women, aged 15 to 29, percentages reporting abortions now peak in the second highest socioeconomic level, whether measured by wife's education, or husband's education or occupation (231, Table 3).

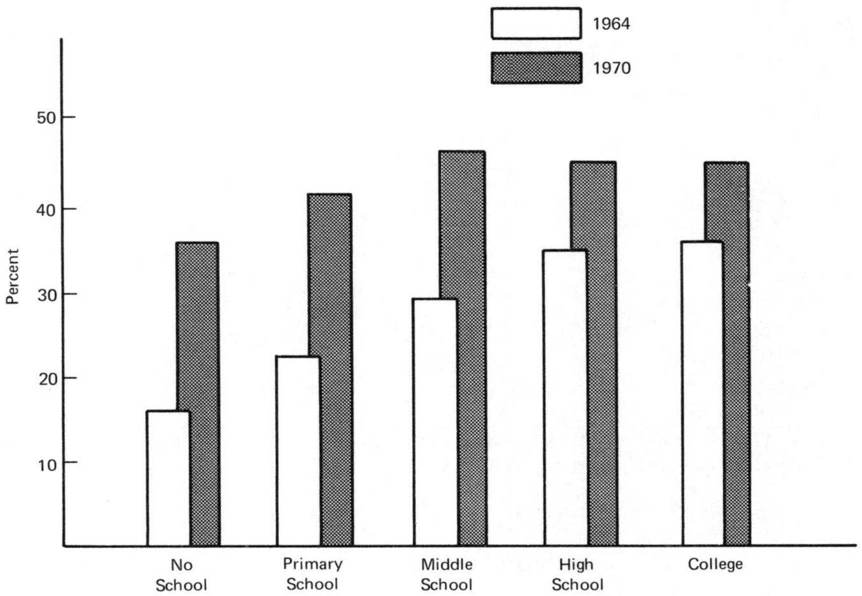

Figure 5-1. Percent of Wives Reporting Induced Abortion, by Educational Level, Songdong-Gu, Seoul, Republic of Korea, 1964 and 1970. Source: S.-B. Hong. *Changing patterns of induced abortion in Seoul, Korea.* Seoul: The Population Council, 1971, figure III-3, p. 31.

Commenting on results of Korea's 1971 Fertility-Abortion Survey, Moon, Han and Choi conclude:

There is a clear tendency for urban women with better education and higher standards of living to rely most on induced abortion. This connotes the potential for urban rates to continue to rise as the population in general and the better-educated population in particular concentrate in urban areas. In addition, the lifetime number of abortions which a woman is likely to have is also increasing. This heralds the idea that women are more and more depending on induced abortion as simply one of a number of tools for birth control. (144, p. 97)

Socioeconomic Development, Infant Mortality, and Desired Family Size. Urbanization, per capita income growth, rises in women's educational levels, and declines in infant mortality occurred rapidly in Korea and Taiwan during the 1960s (see Appendix table), which, together with a tight housing situation in urban areas (Seoul in particular), could be expected to have lowered desired family size and sharpened efforts to control fertility, as in postwar Eastern Europe and Japan. However, desired family size has remained relatively high: 3.8 in Taiwan in 1970 and 3.7 in Korea in 1971. This can be largely attributed to

Table 5-3
Crude Birth Rates, and Abortion, Pill, and IUD Use, by Socioeconomic Level, Seoul, Republic of Korea, 1971

Census Enumeration Districts (ED) by Socioeconomic Status (SES)	Crude Birth Rate for 2 Years, 10 Months Since January 1, 1969	Percent of Ever-Married Women Aged 15-54 Who Have Ever Used		
		Abortion	Pill	IUD
High SES (4 EDs)	17	44	25	17
Average SES (6 EDs)	24	41	22	18
Low SES (6 EDs)	33	31	20	21
Seoul Suburbs (low SES, 4 EDs)	31	33	22	22

Source: W.B. Watson. 1971 fertility-abortion survey quick report No. 17. Seoul: The Population Council, November 5, 1971, table 1.

the continuing common emphasis on the necessity for at least two sons. In both countries there has been a decline since 1965 in the proportion of survey respondents considering three sons as ideal, particularly among women under 30. However, the ideal family size still included 2.1 sons in Taiwan in 1970 and 2.2 in Korea in 1971 (80, 144).

Israel

In Israel, also, abortion is technically illegal in most cases but cheaply and safely available privately from doctors, and appears today to be "one of the most popular methods of family planning used," according to Bachi (13, p. 281). No public family-planning services exist, and modern contraception is relatively unpracticed (82). Among urban Jewish married women surveyed in 1971, 5 percent reportedly used the IUD, 18 percent pills, and 57 percent no contraception (83). (Corresponding percentages for the United States as a whole were 4.5, 22, and 35 percent, according to the 1970 National Fertility Survey. However, in the U.S. survey noncontraceptors consisted mostly of women who were pregnant, trying to get pregnant, in postpartum, or infertile. See Chapter 4.) Abortion is used with varying frequency in the different subpopulation groups, which is associated with differing fertility levels. Surveys of the early 1960s reveal that percentages of women (all ages combined) admitting to at least one abortion among Jewish women were 20.8 for those born in Europe or America (rising to over 50 percent in Tel Aviv-Haifa), 10 for native-born Israeli, and 4.6 for those of African or Asian origin. Only 1.2 percent of Moslem women and 2.7

of the Christians reported previous abortions (13, Table 1). The following data for 1968 were reported to the U.N. Statistical Office (241): medical or legal abortions per 1000 live births: 10 among non-Jews, 62 among Jews; abortions not specified as induced or spontaneous (but presumably induced for the most part, as spontaneous abortion data were given separately) per 1000 births: 76 among non-Jews, 189 among Jews. (In that year the *legal* abortion ratio in Sweden was 96 [58].)

In 1970, the total fertility rate still averaged a high 7.7 per woman among non-Jewish women (mainly Arab), compared to 3.5 among all Jewish women. Jewish women of Afro-Asian origin averaged 4.5, and of European origin, 2.5 (83). (Non-Jews comprised about 17 percent of the total population in 1970 [83].)

Israel's spectacular socioeconomic development since the state's foundation in 1948, high levels of urbanization and female education (see Appendix table), and limited housing could be expected to encourage exceptional efforts to reduce family size, at least among Jews, despite countervailing concerns about ethnic imbalance (far higher Arab fertility) and the need for a substantial population as security against hostile neighbors. Actual family size, even among Jews, does indeed remain somewhat above that of Western industrialized nations.

Latin America

Status of Abortion. The abortion laws of Latin American countries are stringent, normally permitting abortion only for strictly medical reasons, if at all (33). A partial exception is Uruguay, which in principle waives penalties for abortions performed in cases of "serious economic difficulty" (252). Illegal abortion is acknowledged as widespread, however (33, 186, 255). This is viewed as a health problem, the elimination of which has been given as the primary justification for official support of family planning activities in twelve of the twenty Latin American countries (among the twenty-two listed by Nortman [156: 1973, Table 6]) which by 1973 had such policies. (By 1973, only Barbados, Colombia, Dominican Republic, Jamaica, Puerto Rico, and Trinidad and Tobago had official policies to reduce population growth rates. Argentina and Uruguay already have low birth rates and more developed economies.) However, there is evidence that where high birth rates have begun to fall, abortion has played a primary role.

Abortion Levels, Contraceptive Use, and Fertility. In 1964, among married or formerly married women (legally or consensually) aged 20 to 50 surveyed by the Latin American Center for Demography (CELADE) in seven capital cities, the highest abortion rate per 1000 ever pregnant women[a] was found in *Buenos*

[a]This rate measures a woman's chances of aborting a pregnancy once it occurs (186, p. 787).

Aires—246—along with the lowest average number of live births per woman—1.5 (Table 5-4). The women of Buenos Aires then also had the highest level of "contraceptive effectiveness" (for definition see Table 5-4), indicating that women highly motivated to limit family size practice contraception and, when this fails, induce abortion (160, 187).

Abortion ratios are also high in *Uruguay*—an estimated three abortions for each live birth in Montevideo (84, 193), which contains the bulk of the country's population. In both Argentina, of which Buenos Aires is the capital, and Uruguay family-planning programs are very limited (190), but unlike Latin America generally, a high proportion of illegal abortions is safely available from doctors (33, pp. 173-74). Estimated birth rates in these two countries in 1972 were the lowest of all Latin American countries, 22 and 21 per 1000 population respectively (173). (Barbados also stood at 21 per 1000 in that year.) It should be noted, however, that levels of women's education, urbanization, and per capita incomes are at or near the top for the area (Appendix table). Also, unlike other Latin American countries (especially Brazil, Mexico, and Venezuela), a great majority of the population has shared in the substantial benefits of economic and social progress, thus, Rich suggests, ensuring a wider-spread motivation to family limitation (190).

More recent CELADE-conducted or sponsored surveys of abortion, contraception, and fertility of women of all marital statuses, aged 15 to 49, in Bogota, Lima, Panama, and Buenos Aires (36, 85), and in five cities of Paraguay (86) revealed sharply increasing abortion ratios and declining general fertility rates

Table 5-4
Fertility, Contraceptive, and Abortion Characteristics of Ever-Married Women Aged 20-50, in Seven Latin American Capitals, 1964

	Average Number of Live Births per Woman	Abortions (spontaneous and induced) per 1,000 Ever-Pregnant Women	Level of Contraceptive Effectiveness[a]
Mexico City	3.3	155	13.7
Bogota	3.2	117	21.8
San Jose of Costa Rica	3.0	161	27.2
Caracas	3.0	163	24.4
Panama	2.7	211	
Rio de Janeiro	2.3	141	
Buenos Aires	1.5	246	41.8

[a]Level of contraceptive effectiveness was computed by adding the percent of women using effective contraceptives in each city and the percent who used ineffective contraceptives multiplied by 0.50.

Source: M. Requena. The problem of induced abortion in Latin America. *Demography*, 1968, 5, table 1, p. 790.

over the five-year period preceding the surveys in Bogota, Lima, and Panama (Table 5-5).[b] Numbers of pregnancies (abortions plus live births) per 1000 women had also fallen in these three cities, especially in Bogota, indicating that contraception was also being increasingly used to control fertility. However, abortion appears still to carry the greater weight—most markedly in Lima, where the abortion ratio for the year preceding the survey rose 85 percent over the average for the four years before that, while the pregnancy rate fell 12 percent and the fertility rate dropped 22 percent.

In *Buenos Aires*, according to this 1969 survey, abortion was down and fertility up, but underreporting of abortion is suspected here, and since Buenos Aires' fertility level had been low for many years (and was lowest of the five cities at the time of these surveys), Carrasco suggests that the apparent rise "might be the result of occasional fluctuations in fertility" (36).

Separate data for *Asuncion* from the Paraguayan five-city study show an 85 percent increase in annual abortions per 1000 pregnancies, a slight drop in pregnancy rates (not specified), and a 44 percent drop in fertility rates for the decade preceding the 1971 survey, in contrast to the rises of 16 percent in the abortion/pregnancy ratio and 4 percent in general fertility rates for the five-year period seen in Table 5-5 (86, Chapter 11). In Asuncion in 1970-71, a quarter of the lifetime average of 4.5 pregnancies per woman were aborted, and the crude birth rate had dropped to the moderate level of 29 per 1000 population (86), in contrast to an estimated 45 per 1000 for the country as a whole (239). Official family planning had begun in Paraguay shortly before this survey, but was still confined to Asuncion and one or two other cities (86).

Gaslonde and Carrasco, authors of the study reviews on which Tables 5-5 and 7-1 are based, found a lower incidence of abortion among users of more effective contraceptive methods. They conclude from this and other evidence that the increasing use of pills, injections, IUDs, and sterilization obtained largely through family-planning programs recently begun in all the cities surveyed except Lima has been more effective in reducing the incidence of abortion—the declared objective of the programs—than in checking or diminishing fertility. (However, at the time of the surveys these modern contraceptive methods were

[b]In these CELADE-sponsored studies and those of 1964, women were asked only about "abortions" experienced. It was felt this would elicit more truthful reporting of total abortions than a direct attempt to inquire about spontaneous and induced abortions separately. Estimates of induced abortions were subsequently derived by assuming on the basis of independent evidence that a constant proportion of all pregnancies end in spontaneous abortions. The 1964 surveys set this constant proportion as between 80 and 100 per 1000 pregnancies (186), while the more recent surveys assumed a fixed proportion of 100 in every 1000 pregnancies (36, 85). Data shown in Tables 5-4, 5-5, and 7-1 are based on total abortions reported. Thus, these abortion rates and ratios cannot be compared with those quoted elsewhere in this book. However, trends in induced abortion can be derived—assuming constant levels of spontaneous abortions. But it should be noted that in some cases abortion ratios fall below 100 per 1000 pregnancies (e.g., among women with three or more previous live births in Table 7-1), suggesting that among such women there is no induced abortion (at least reported), and a below-average level of spontaneous abortion.

Table 5-5

Trends in Abortion Ratios, Pregnancy Rates, and General Fertility Rates in the Five Years Preceding Each Survey Among Women Aged 15-44, Bogota, Lima, Panama, Buenos Aires, Asuncion

		Abortions[a] per 1,000 Pregnancies			Pregnancies per 1,000 Women			Live Births per 1,000 Women		
	Year of Survey	Preceding Year	Four Years Before That	Percent Change[b]	Preceding Year	Four Years Before That	Percent Change[b]	Preceding Year	Four Years Before That	Percent Change[b]
Bogota	1968	147	115	+28	119	143	−17	101	126	−20
Lima	1970	227	123	+85	142	123	−12	109	139	−22
Panama	1969	192	165	+16	138	144	− 4	108	118	− 8
Buenos Aires	1969	188	217	−13	99	88	+13	79	67	+18
Asuncion	1971	223	192	+16	148	139	+ 6	114	110	+ 4

[a]Including spontaneous and induced.

[b]Percent change in rates of the year preceding each survey from the average annual rates during the four years prior to that.

Source: E. Carrasco. Incidence of abortion, fertility and contraception in Latin America, in International Union for the Scientific Study of Population, *International Population Conference, Liège, 1973*, Vol. 2, Liège: Author, 1973, table 1, p. 309.

used by less than 10 percent of women interviewed in Lima and Asuncion, although by 24 percent of women in Panama [85]. No data are given for Bogota.) Abortion has had the greater weight in the recent fertility declines (with the probable exception of Buenos Aires, where fertility is already low) because of its great increase among older women, aged 35 to 44. Abortion rates had actually declined among younger women, aged 20 to 34 except in Lima. From this it would appear that abortion is being used increasingly in at least these capital cities as a means to limit, if not space, fertility (36, 85, 86). In Santiago, Chile, a more detailed prospective study (also sponsored by CELADE) of 804 married women interviewed thirteen times at monthly intervals between October 1969 and December 1970 disclosed highest abortion rates among the youngest (25 to 29) nonemployed women, and "middle-aged" (30 to 34) working women (202). This suggests that in Santiago, at least, induced abortion is being used by young women "just starting families" to space births, as well as older working women to limit family size (probably because their employment is essential to supplement family income).

Conning includes Chile (capital: Santiago), Colombia (capital: Bogota), Panama, and Peru (capital: Lima) among eleven Latin American countries where fertility has apparently declined since 1960, while crude birth rates appear to have stabilized in Paraguay (capital: Asuncion). In all cases declines appear to have started before launching of government-sponsored or -assisted national family-planning programs, suggesting that *social and economic changes* have been more instrumental in precipitating such declines. In searching for significant explanatory socioeconomic indicators, he finds no correlation between fertility trends and changes in per capita income and life expectancy. The most significant association is between fertility decline and higher percentages of 15 to 19-year olds in secondary school (47). From the Appendix table it can be seen that in Chile, Colombia, Panama, and Peru—and Argentina (though not Paraguay)—over 20 percent of eligible females were enrolled in secondary schools by the late 1960s, in contrast to, for instance, only 16 and 20 percent respectively in Mexico and Brazil, where no drop in fertility had occurred. Also, except for Paraguay, over half or nearly half of the population was urbanized. However, Conning concludes from his (admittedly limited) investigation that no single set of socioeconomic indicators can explain fertility decline in every case.

Chile. Extensive surveys in Chile (chiefly sponsored by CELADE) provide the best information to study the relationship between *incidence of induced abortion, use of contraception, and fertility trends* in Latin America.

In Chile, hospital admissions for treatment of incomplete abortions rose from 84 to 204 per 1000 deliveries between 1937 and 1964 (160, Table 3), to 234 in 1966, with a slight drop to 212 in 1968 (182, Chapter 11). Deliveries increased 1.8 times in these years, whereas postabortion hospital admissions went up 4.4 times. (The rise in abortion admissions may be due to an increased tendency to seek medical attention for all types of disorders or emergencies, but this should apply also to deliveries/childbirth.) In 1962, Plaza and Briones estimated that as a result of abortion complications some 45,800 Chilean women were hospitalized for 150,000 bed-days, at a cost of over 1 million dollars (170). The actual incidence of abortion is, of course, much higher. (Armijo and Monreal estimated that in the early 1960s about one-third of induced illegal abortions in Santiago led to hospitalization [11].) A 1959 survey of 2000 women in Santiago found an abortion ratio of 1 to 3 live births for legally married women and 1 to slightly over 2 for consensually or formerly married and separated women (222). Separate surveys in Santiago in 1962-63 estimated that between 16.6 and 23.4 percent of all pregnancies terminated in *induced* abortion (10, 186). (In 1970, a retrospective survey of 675 married women, conducted in association with the prospective survey mentioned above, produced an estimate of 20.7 percent of all pregnancies terminating in induced abortion, which falls within the range of these similar earlier Santiago surveys. However, the prospective survey produced an estimate of 33.6 percent, which suggests that estimates of the prevalence of induced abortion based on one-time retrospective interviews are subject to respondents' faulty recall and/or deliberate underreporting, and may yield estimates up to 50 percent lower than actual prevalence [202].) In one study, only a quarter of women aged 20 to 44 were practicing contraception, including abstinence (10). The Chilean recorded crude birth rate dropped only slightly from 34.6 to 32.8 between 1936 and 1964; less than might be expected, in view of the rising incidence of abortion in these years. However, it is suggested that underreporting of births in earlier years and increasing proportions of fertile women—due to improved health conditions—probably mask a real decline in fertility, which is unreflected in crude birth rates (160), so that it seems plausible, as Requena and Monreal argue (188), that had it not been for abortion, Chilean birth rates in these years would have been over 40 per 1000 population for the whole country and over 50 for the lower socioeconomic groups.

Organized family planning was introduced into Santiago in 1963 and to the rest of the country in 1964 (188). Between 1963 and 1967 the percentage of fertile-aged women in Santiago protected by pills and IUDs (including those obtained outside the program) rose from 0.4 to 13 (143). Two comparable surveys in the city in 1962 and 1967 revealed that in this period there had been a drop of 27.5 points in the fertility rate (198.7 to 171.2 births per 1000 women aged 20 to 44), and an *increase* of 11.6 points in the rate of induced abortions (44.7 to 56.5 abortions per 1000 women [143, Table 10]). The ratio of induced abortions per 1000 pregnancies also rose in the surveyed populations—from 155 to 201 (143, Table 9). Monreal and Armijo concluded from these studies that births averted after 1963 were prevented approximately half by contraception available through the family-planning program and half by increased abortion. By 1970-72, Chile's estimated crude birth rate of 28-30 per 1000 (173, 239) was among Latin America's lowest. Conning calculates that crude birth rates and general fertility rates fell by some 30 percent in Chile during the 1960s, with particularly sharp fertility declines after 1965 among women aged 30 and over (47).

Changing Socioeconomic Differentials in Abortion, Contraceptive Use, and Fertility in Latin America. This 1962-67 Santiago study also seemed to confirm Requena's hypothesis that social classes in a community or nation, as well as nations as a whole, progress through three stages in the complementary use of abortion and contraception as they move through the demographic transition from high to low fertility (187) in response to socioeconomic progress or organized family planning (Figure 1-1). Studies in the early and mid-1960s in Santiago, Colombia, Costa Rica, Mexico, and Brazil suggest that however socioeconomic status is measured (education, income, husband or wife's occupation), in the period that countries are just beginning to take off socioeconomically and before the initiation of organized family planning, the lowest social classes have the least incidence of contraceptive use and abortion and highest fertility rates, while the reverse is true of upper classes, with "middle-class" women having the highest incidence of abortion (4, 5, 7, 90, 187, 259). However, between 1962 and 1967 in Santiago induced abortion rates went up substantially among the lowest classes (from 32 to 53 per 1000 "lower-middle level" women, and 49 to 75 per 1000 "lower-lower" women), and dropped from 37 to 25 per 1000 women classified as "upper and upper-middle level" (143, Table 11). At the same time, the general fertility rate declined 33 percent in the lowest classes and increased slightly in the "lower-middle" and upper classes. Monreal and Armijo concluded that the family-planning program had stimulated "an awakening to the necessity for limiting the family in many marginal sectors" (143), which is first satisfied by the "curative" use of abortion rather than the "preventive" use of contraception (187, p. 350). (Monreal and Armijo hint that the preference for abortion over contraception to meet the awakened fertility-control desires of Santiago's lowest classes may have been partially due to inadequate and inconveniently located sources of contraceptive advice and supplies in the early years of the program.) In the later 1969-70 Santiago studies, highest abortion rates were also found among women of the lowest class (202).

In the Appendix table it can be seen that about 1970, Chile's per capita income (GNP) was well below that of Venezuela (U.S. $720 compared to U.S. $980), the percentage of eligible women enrolled in secondary school no more (36 versus 37 percent), and infant mortality rates still close to 60 percent higher than in Venezuela (79 compared to 50 deaths per 1000 live births), and yet Chile's crude birth rate had fallen substantially by this time, while Venezuela's remained above 40 per 1000 population. This suggests that, in addition to socioeconomic development, the organized family-planning program was a prime factor in arousing the desire for family limitation in Chile, by whatever means available. Family planning has received strong government support in Chile since 1966, but only since 1972 in Venezuela (156: 1973, Table 6).

Since the lowest classes are most numerous (certainly in Latin America), it is suggested that this shift down the social scale in maximum incidence of abortion will probably increase the total number of abortions (182, Chapter 11), and presumably mean that abortion has a greater impact than contraception in lowering national fertility rates in the initial stages of organized family planning or as the benefits of socioeconomic development also begin to move down the social scale, arousing in their wake the desire to limit (or even space) children. In the more recent five-capital studies, the lowest classes–measured by women's education–exhibited the highest abortion rates; except, surprisingly, in Buenos Aires, most economically advanced of the cities (85, Table 2).

Rural-Urban Differentials. Similarly, the rural-urban pattern in Latin America with respect to abortion, fertility, and contraception suggests an initially greater impact of abortion in lowering fertility rates.

In *Colombia* by 1967 the general fertility rate in rural areas was 210 compared to 130 per 1000 women in urban areas; the abortion rates were two to four times lower in all income groups compared to similar rates in urban areas; and it is estimated that in rural areas only a small percentage of potential pregnancies were averted by contraception (4, Table 19A and Figure 4. This figure shows a higher contraceptive use and lower abortion rates in Bogota, the largest city, than in medium-sized cities).

In *Chile*, in the early 1960s, the percentage of women with one or more induced abortions was 35 in the capital, Santiago, and went down to 7 in La Calera, a predominantly rural community 100 kilometers from Santiago (186). The risk of induced abortion was lower for women who had lived less than ten years in the city than for those who had lived there at least ten years (133 compared to 260 induced abortions per 1000 ever-pregnant women respectively). A rural-urban comparative fertility study of this period found an average of 2.5 children, per woman interviewed in Santiago, compared to 4.2 and 5.0 in two "rural-small urban" areas in Chile (142, Table 2).

Viel is certain that rapid urbanization in Latin America during the 1960s (see Appendix table) has inevitably provoked an overall increase in abortion (256). This in turn should eventually contribute to declines in national rates of fertility. (However, there is evidence in Latin America of narrowing rural-urban differentials in fertility. This may be due to a lag in adoption of both contraception and abortion and consequently undiminished fertility among recently arrived rural immigrants in large cities, who form an increasingly large proportion of total city population. See Salazar, 201; Weller et al., 265; and Zarate, 272.)

6 Impact of Intensive Family Planning Programs on Abortion and Fertility (Chile, Japan, Republic of Korea)

Experimental family-planning programs in Chile, Japan, and Korea demonstrate that with intensive input it is possible to lower fertility with no—or a shortened—intervening period of increased abortion.

In the *San Gregorio area of Santiago* a program stressing IUDs was begun in March 1965. By the end of 1966, 16 percent of women of childbearing age were protected by the program, in contrast to 8-10 percent in the surrounding Southern Health area of the city, where a general family-planning program had begun five years earlier. The general fertility rate had dropped 22 percent since 1964, the year prior to the special program's start, and the abortion rate also dropped by 40 percent (73), in contrast to the abortion increase in the city generally in this period, as already noted.

In *Japan* during the 1950s, six communities received intensive family-planning advice and supplies (all methods except pills and IUDs). Crude birth rates dropped from 27.4 in the year before the programs began to 10.0 per 1000 in the fifth year of "guidance." The abortion rate also dropped from 8.7 to 3.7 per 1000 women by the fifth year, but only after a rise in the early years, which Koya attributes to the population's initial contraceptive inexperience and consequent high failure rates (125).

In *Korea* in 1963-64, marital fertility fell by 38 percent in one township subjected to an experimental family-planning program (also excluding IUDs and pills), compared to 13 percent in a neighboring township exposed to only the routine government program. This appears to have been due to a better use of contraceptives, rather than a more extensive use of abortion or abortion plus contraception (Sook Bang, 1968, cited in 182, Chapter 11).

The high costs and numbers of personnel involved in these concentrated programs would make such intensive efforts difficult at the national level. Requena remarks: "Even if the necessary resources and personnel were available, their employment cannot be justified compared with the priorities presented by other public health programs" (187, p. 351).

7 Recently Observed Levels of Abortion by Age, Marital Status and Previous Live Births

Increasing Abortion Among Teenagers

Data on legal abortions collected by Tietze and Dawson for eleven countries[a] with such statistics and New York City, and on all induced abortions in the Republic of Korea, show that the great majority of abortions (70-90 percent) and the highest age-specific abortion rates (annual numbers of abortions per 1000 women aged 19 or less, 20-24, 25-29, 30-34, 35-39, or 40 or more) occur among women aged 20 to 39 (231, p. 5, Tables 4 and 5). This is to be expected, since this age span encompasses the greatest amount of sexual and family-building activity. However, these data also show that over the period for which data are available the proportion of women under 20 among all aborters has been increasing—reaching 22-29 percent in the United States, England and Wales, Scotland, and Sweden for the latest year given (1971 or 1972), and almost 33 percent in the state of California, although it is still less than 3 percent in Singapore and Japan. Also, increases in age-specific abortion rates over the periods covered have been greater in this than in any other age group. In Sweden the abortion rate for women aged 19 or less has actually been highest of all age groups since 1968. In 1971 it stood at 16.8 abortions per 1000, fourteen times the 1956 rate of 1.2, and more than four times the rate of 3.8 in 1965, when the more permissive official abortion practices began. (However, in the same year the comparable figure for Hungary was 37.1.)

In Latin America, also, the increase in induced abortion (although illegal) has apparently been greatest among the very youngest women. In Bogota, Lima, Buenos Aires, and Asuncion the ratio of abortions (spontaneous plus induced) to pregnancies in the year just prior to the recent surveys had increased more in relation to the preceding four years among 15- to 19-year-old women than in the 20-34 or 35-44 age groups. The rise was particularly marked in Bogota and Lima. In the first city abortion ratios went up 117 percent among youngest women (42 to 91 abortions per 1000 pregnancies), compared to 11 percent among women aged 20 to 34 (124 to 138), and 78 percent among the oldest women surveyed (135 to 240). In Lima the rises were 162 percent among youngest women (127 to 333), 98 percent among the middle group (108 to 214), and 31 percent among the oldest women (191 to 250). In Panama the increase among youngest women was as great as that among the oldest (36, Table 1).

[a]Czechoslovakia, Denmark, England and Wales, Finland, Hungary, Japan, Scotland, Singapore, Sweden, United States, and Yugoslavia.

Increases Among the Unmarried

Abortion is also increasing among the unmarried, according to Tietze and Dawson's data. Although among the countries listed (231, Table 9) the majority of legal aborters are currently married in all but the United States, Sweden, and England and Wales, the balance is shifting, and everywhere but in Sweden abortion ratios have increased most among the unmarried during the time periods covered (231, Table 10). In Santiago, Chile, also, abortion rates (although it is not clear if ratios or rates are meant) increased more among the unmarried than the married between the surveys of 1962 and 1967 (143, Table 13).

Tietze and Dawson remark that the "apparently world-wide and rapid increase in the rates of legal abortions among young women may reflect early maturation, changing patterns of sexual behavior [and] growing acceptance of abortion as an alternative to forced motherhood" (231, p. 27), developments that would apply also to the unmarried (composed largely of the never married). These developments may also be associated with the similar increases noted among youngest women in at least the five Latin American capital cities surveyed recently, where abortion is still illegal. Liberalization of abortion laws and accompanying changes in medical attitudes and practices may also encourage increased resort to abortion among young and/or unmarried women confronted with unplanned pregnancies. This is suggested by the fact that among Zelnik and Kantner's national sample of 4611 umarried teenaged women surveyed in the United States in 1971 "very few" of the currently or formerly pregnant had had or contemplated an abortion (273). (The original sample included about 10 percent married teenagers, but analysis so far published has been based only on the unmarried.) At this time legal abortion had only just become available in a limited number of states. Presumably the high and increasing proportions of the young and unmarried noted among aborters in those areas where abortion had been liberalized by 1971 (see especially New York City, California, and Washington state, above) forecast a trend for the United States as a whole as legal abortion becomes readily available in the wake of the January 1973 Supreme Court decisions (provided these are not overturned by the increasing pressure for a Constitutional amendment). It has also been seen that legalization of abortion appears to have increased the tendency (and the possibility) for young, unmarried British women to seek abortion.

Cutright has noted that in less than a decade following legalization of abortion on request annual rates of illegitimacy dropped by up to 50 percent in Hungary, Czechoslovakia, and Poland, and illegitimacy was all but eliminated by 1965 in Japan. This suggests that complete liberalization of abortion elsewhere could have a similar rapid impact on illegitimacy. Cutright notes: "There is no evidence from any population that such a decline in an illegitimacy rate can be achieved with a contraception-only program" (49, p. 425).

It has frequently been suggested, implicitly or explicitly, that liberal abortion attitudes have given rise to the increasing numbers of unplanned pregnancies among the young unmarried as well as their increased tendency to seek abortion once such pregnancies occur. There are no data to refute or support this suggestion, but some clues suggest that the relationship is not causal. For example, premarital pregnancy *rates* (numbers of premaritally conceived births per 1000 women aged 15 to 44) have risen in New Zealand where the abortion law is restrictive, as well as in England where it is permissive (180)—although actual numbers of premaritally conceived births fell in England after 1968 to at least 1971, as noted in Chapter 4.

Parity

Corresponding to the increase in abortions among the young and unmarried, the proportion of aborters with no (or only one) prior birth has also been increasing in countries with legal abortion for which Tietze and Dawson provide data (231, Table 7). In recent years, proportions of childless women among legal aborters have been highest in the United States (51 percent), England and Wales (46 percent), and Sweden (41 percent). Proportions of women with only one prior birth have been highest in Czechoslovakia (21 percent) and Hungary (33 percent). In Japan, 22.3 percent of respondents in the 1969 nationwide survey reported that they had aborted their first pregnancy (172). These are all economically developed countries where evidently legal abortion is being increasingly used (where contraception fails or has been neglected) to postpone first births especially, and to space early births, as well as limit overall family size in response to rising exigencies of city living and heightened female educational and occupational expectations (33, Chapter 8). In Singapore, however, only 1 percent of the women aborted in 1972 were childless, while 40 percent had experienced at least five births, indicating that here abortion is still seen primarily as a means of family limitation rather than spacing.

Tietze and Dawson point out that the number of prior births at which the abortion ratio (abortions per 1000 births) is highest corresponds to the number of children beyond which additional births become unacceptable to a substantial proportion of women (231, p. 28). According to the data presented (231, Table 8), this is evidently two or three prior births in Czechoslovakia and Hungary, and three or four in Finland and the United States, although in the latter two countries abortion ratios are also relatively high among childless women and lowest among those with only one prior birth. However, in Korea and Singapore abortion ratios climb steadily from women without prior births to those of the highest parity. The researchers explain this as indicating that the small family norm is relatively new in these countries, and therefore women of high parity do not here represent a group selected for rejection of abortion.

Table 7-1

Lifetime Abortion Ratios and Rates According to Previous Live Births at Time of the Survey Among Women Aged 20-49, Bogota, Lima, Panama, and Buenos Aires, 1968-70

	Bogota		Lima		Panama		Buenos Aires	
Previous Live Births at Time of Survey	Abortion Ratio[a]	Abortion Rate[b]	Abortion Ratio	Abortion Rate	Abortion Ratio	Abortion Rate	Abortion Ratio	Abortion Rate
1	174	213	190	259	236	324	240	333
2	121	277	128	298	147	355	163	396
3	92	307	118	406	117	405	236	935
4	108	486	93	417	108	495	111	508
5 or more	91	663	78	568	98	722	124	873

[a]Number of abortions (spontaneous and induced) to date of survey per 1,000 pregnancies.

[b]Number of abortions (spontaneous and induced) to date per 1,000 women surveyed.

Source: S. Gaslonde. Abortion-fertility studies in Asuncion, Bogota, Buenos Aires, Lima, and Panama. In H.P. David and S. Cambiaso (eds.), *Abortion and family planning practices in Latin America.* Washington: Pan American Health Organization, 1974, forthcoming, table 6.

Curiously, in four of the Latin American capitals recently surveyed by CELADE (Asuncion was omitted from this particular analysis) the ratios of abortions to pregnancies (abortions plus live births) were highest among women with only one prior birth (Table 7-1; no data were given for childless women). The data in Table 7-1 cover the lifetime experience to date of all women interviewed, so that it is to be expected that abortion *rates* (numbers of previous abortions per 1000 women interviewed) climb with increasing parity. The more live births (and pregnancies) a woman has had, the greater her chances of having resorted to abortion. However, in Buenos Aires the abortion rate is highest among women with three prior births—more than double the rate of women with two previous births (935 compared to 396 abortions per 1000 women interviewed). This suggests that a moderate-sized family of three children has become the norm in this most developed of the four capital cities.

While contraception rather than abortion is to be encouraged among the young, the unmarried, and/or the childless to avert unplanned pregnancies, it is evident that when such pregnancies do occur the women concerned are increasingly resorting to abortion. Legalization of abortion appears to facilitate this possibility, particularly as countries reach higher stages of socioeconomic development. As suggested in the introduction, this may prove to be the greatest contribution legalization of abortion might make to long-run population trends, in addition to the humanitarian and social aspects of consequently reduced numbers of out-of-wedlock births, unwanted children, interrupted educational and occupational plans, and too early, forced marriage.

8 Summary and Conclusions

By early 1974, abortion on request in the first three months of pregnancy, or for social, economic, or broadly defined physical and mental health reasons was legally available in some twenty-seven countries, containing over half the world's population. These liberal laws have been enacted in a desire to reduce the costly personal and societal ill effects of widely practiced illegal abortion and to ensure women the right to complete control of their own fertility. Nowhere has control of population growth been an explicitly expressed official motive (with the possible exception of the People's Republic of China, Singapore, and Tunisia). Nor is induced abortion advocated as a substitute for effective contraception in any attempt to reduce rates of population growth. Yet the question arises to what extent legalization and wide availability of safe, early abortion, in conjunction with freely available modern contraception, might accelerate the process of fertility decline in developing countries and the attainment of replacement fertility levels in developed countries.

This volume has summarized some of the available evidence in an attempt to answer this question.

Fertility trends were reviewed following the abrupt change from restrictive to de jure and de facto permissive abortion in Japan (1948), Eastern Europe and the U.S.S.R. (1955-60), New York City (July 1970), and, as far as possible, the People's Republic of China (intermittently since 1957); and also following official restriction of permissive abortion in Bulgaria, Czechoslovakia, and Romania. Trends were noted subsequent to relatively more moderate legal changes in Great Britain (1967), Singapore (1969), California, Maryland, and Washington state (1967-70), and in Scandinavia, where long-standing moderate abortion laws have recently been extended or interpreted more liberally. Fertility trends were also noted where abortion has been or is still technically illegal but evidently widely practiced: the Republic of Korea, Taiwan, Western Europe, Israel (Jewish population), Latin America, and the United States and Great Britain before 1967.

In examining these fertility trends an attempt has been made to ascertain the degree to which abortion is available in practice as well as law; of the nature and extent of concurrent contraceptive practice; and of the extent to which legal abortions following liberalization simply replace abortions which would have occurred with no changes in the law. Also, where relevant, brief account was taken of other important factors that bear upon observed fertility trends: changes in ages at marriage and in sexual behavior; in the age-sex and rural-urban structure of the population; and, most important, the concurrent socioeconomic situation and levels of infant mortality, which largely determine the *motivation* to fertility control, for which contraception and induced abortion normally serve only as the means.

The most dramatic recorded declines in fertility over relatively short time periods appear to have generally occurred where elective abortion has been introduced to a population already strongly motivated to control family size and practicing only traditional or no contraception at the time of legalization: Eastern Europe, the U.S.S.R., Japan, and, according to some reports, the People's Republic of China, where free abortion and contraception were introduced and made widely available simultaneously in at least the two most recent birth control campaigns: 1962-66 and 1969 to the present. Over time, birth rates have leveled or declined more slowly in these countries, but the weight in fertility control has shifted from abortion to contraception (with the possible exception of the U.S.S.R.) as contraception becomes more widespread and more effective contraceptives have been adopted, although the availability of ready abortion may have somewhat retarded the adoption of pills and IUDs in Eastern Europe.

Marked fertility declines have also occurred following introduction of legal and widely available abortion in developed areas presumably already practicing modern contraception: New York City, California, Maryland, Washington state, and possibly Great Britain. This has evidently been due in part to the wide use of legal abortion to terminate unplanned and undesired pregnancies among groups where contraception is unpracticed or less efficient and for whom safe abortion was previously less accessible—black women in the United States, and particularly the young and the unmarried. Where abortion has been legalized in the United States, subsequent abortion levels have been higher and fertility declines usually greater among black women than among whites; and in both the United States and Great Britain legal abortion is apparently "keeping a lid" on what otherwise would be a continuation of previously accelerating rises in numbers of out-of-wedlock and premaritally conceived births and teenage "shotgun" marriages. Even where it is assumed that contraception is now practiced almost universally at least by the married, evidence from the United States and Great Britain indicates that the use of ineffective methods and contraceptive risk-taking are more widespread and resulting unplanned pregnancies more frequent than would be expected. For the United States it is estimated that adoption of legal abortion on a national scale equivalent to that observed in New York City since July 1970 could avert most of the births now estimated as unplanned and consequently reduce national birth rates to near replacement levels.

It is evident in at least New York City, California, and Singapore that legalization of abortion does not encourage contraceptive laxity among women already practicing efficient contraception.

Owing to its clandestine nature, the extent of illegal abortion can only be estimated by indirect means. Therefore, it is impossible to gauge with accuracy by how much legal abortions following upon law changes more than replace prior illegal abortions and hence have a net impact on subsequent fertility trends. Because birth rates in the 1930s were as low as—or little higher than—those now current in, for example, Great Britain and Scandinavia (with the exception of Finland), it would seem that in Western industrialized countries legalization has resulted mainly in a substitution of legal for illegal abortion with little, if any, long-term impact on fertility trends (though considerable impact as a health measure). However, short-term fertility declines in these countries have been associated with changes in abortion laws and practice compressed into relatively brief time periods. In many cases, "guestimates" of annual numbers of illegal abortion prior to legalization vary widely, which further complicates the attempt to measure the demographic impact of abortion legalization.

A combination of illegal abortions and contraception in restrictive countries that are motivated to control fertility—whether through socioeconomic progress or institution of organized family planning—also helps to reduce fertility rates. The incidence of abortion, although illegal, rose in Taiwan and the Republic of Korea during the 1960s along with increasing use of IUDs, pills, and sterilization supplied through national family planning programs or commercial channels, and is credited with a large share of concurrent birth-rate declines of some 30 percent.

Relatively low birth rates in the United States and Great Britain in the 1930s, and again in Western Europe today, have perhaps been due more to illegal abortion than to the use of effective contraception. In some parts of Western Europe, despite introduction of pills and IUDs, traditional and less reliable methods of contraception seem still to be most common, with increasingly safe and available—though still illegal—abortion used as a backstop. In The Netherlands, as in Korea and Taiwan, the introduction of pills and IUDs seems to have reinforced the desire to avert unplanned births. Unexpected recent declines in fertility are associated with a marked increase in abortions performed by doctors despite continuing legal restrictions.

In Latin America there is evidence that where the desire to limit family size has been aroused, either as the benefits of socioeconomic development have begun to spread to the general population or as organized family planning has been initiated, the incidence of abortion has risen along with increasing use of contraception and is also associated with declines in fertility.

In Romania, Bulgaria, and Czechoslovakia low birth and high abortion rates have prompted official restriction of legal abortion, but after an initial sharp rise, birth rates declined in all three countries, despite continuing de jure restrictions on abortion. (Elective abortion in Hungary was somewhat restricted in January 1974, but it is too early to observe how this might affect that country's fertility.)

It is evident that only very broad legal changes, requiring no bureaucratic involvement and accompanied by full medical and public acceptance, successfully eliminate illegal abortion following legalization.

Although in most countries the majority of aborters tend to be married women (including the consensually mated, as in Latin America), aged 20 to 39, anxious to limit family size, there is worldwide evidence that very young, unmarried, and/or childless women, confronted with unplanned pregnancies, are increasingly resorting to abortion to avert out-of-wedlock births and/or postpone first births. Legalization of abortion appears to facilitate this trend. By lengthening the generation span and increasing the likelihood of lower completed family size, this development potentially reduces the absolute size and growth rate of the population in the future as well as current rates of growth.

Social classes (whether measured by education, occupation, or rural-urban residence), as well as nations, appear to move through three stages in their demographic transition from high to low rates of fertility (and mortality): from no birth prevention and high birth rates, to falling birth rates accomplished primarily by abortion, to low birth rates achieved mainly by contraception, with some residual abortion to meet contraceptive failure. It has been argued that nations tend to progress through these three stages regardless of the legal status of abortion. However, it also appears that, assuming a strong motivation for family limitation, legalized abortion, with a wide range of indications, freely interpreted and readily available, can accelerate this progression.

Experimental family-planning programs in small areas of Chile, Japan, and Korea have indicated that the intervening period of increased abortion can be eliminated or shortened, but that this requires a costly, intensive effort that is probably not feasible or justifiable on a national scale.

Theoretical research demonstrates that, even when consistently used, all presently reversible methods of contraception are not sufficiently reliable in themselves to keep lifetime family size within the two-three children ideal now almost universal in developed countries and hoped for in developing countries. Also, abortion used alone is an inefficient method of fertility regulation, but becomes progressively more efficient as the expanding use of contraception relegates its role to a backstop measure. It takes two to three abortions to avert one birth in a noncontracepting population, but only slightly more than one in a population practicing relatively effective contraception.

While the evidence presented cannot be claimed as conclusive, it appears to be compatible with the conclusion that, on balance, the most effective approach to bringing about a voluntary reduction in high birth rates or reducing moderate birth rates to replacement levels—providing the motivation for fertility control exists—would be a combination of strong contraceptive programs and widely available legal, or condoned, abortion. This policy would also be least costly to maternal health, and possibly in the long run would also be associated with least total induced abortion.

Simple, safe abortion procedures easily adaptable to use by paramedical personnel on an outpatient basis, such as vacuum aspiration in the first three months of pregnancy, could reduce the need for an elaborate medical infrastructure and thus enable developing countries to more adequately meet the demand for abortion following legalization, as appears to be the case in the People's Republic of China.

Appendix Table

Appendix Table
Selected Demographic, Social, and Economic Characteristics for Selected Developed and Developing Countries, with or without Legal Abortion, Selected Years, 1950-72

Developed Countries with Legal Abortion (Year Legalized)	Births per 1,000 Population		Women as % of Total Labor Force		% of All Women in Labor Force		% of Women Aged 15-49 in Labor Force		% of Eligible Women in Secondary School		% Urban of Total Population	
	Year	Rate	Year	%	Year	%	Year	%	Year	%	Year	%
Eastern Europe												
Bulgaria (1956)	1950-54	21.7	1955	30[a]							1950	28
	1960	17.8	1960	34	1965	46	1965	75	1965	65	1960	38
	1971	16.0	1967	41							1970	53
Czecho-slovakia (1957)	1950-54	22.0	1955	37[a]					1960	34	1950	52
	1960	15.9	1960	41	1961	38	1961	63	1965	43	1960	57
	1972	15.3	1967	45	1970	42	1970	73	1969	43	1970	63
German Democratic Republic (1965, 1973)	1950-54	17.0	1955	42[a]							1950	71
	1960	17.2	1960	46	1964	40					1960	72
	1972	11.7	1967	49							1970	74
Hungary (1956)	1950-54	21.1	1955	34[a]					1960	29	1950	38
	1960	14.7	1960	35	1960	33	1960	51	1965	41	1960	42
	1972	14.7	1967	39	1970	39	1970	65	1969	52	1968	47
Poland (1956)	1950-54	30.1	1955	33[a]					1960	42	1950	37
	1960	22.6	1960	33	1960	40	1960	63	1965	53	1960	48
	1972	17.4	1967	37					1969	54	1970	52

[a]Women as percent of total employment in the socialized nonagricultural branches.
[b]Urban
[c]Rural

GNP Per Capita in US $		Average Annual Growth Rate of Per Capita GNP	Infant Deaths per 1,000 Live Births		Average Ideal/ Desired Family Size		Status of Organized Family Planning or Availability of Pill and IUD
Year	Amount	1960-70 %	Year	Rate	Year	Av.	Comment
1970	760	7.4	1964 1970	33 27	1965	1.9	Official contraceptive advice widely available since 1968. Pills imported.
1970	2,230	3.8	1965 1971	26 22	1958-59 1966 1967	2.4 1.9[b] 2.1[c]	Contraceptive advice technically required after delivery/childbirth since 1958. Pills and IUDs manufactured.
1970	2,490	4.2	1964 1970	29 19			Official family planning since 1966. Pills and IUDs widely available since mid-1960s.
1970	1,600	5.4	1964 1970	40 36	1958-60 1965-66	2.3 2.1	Pills available since 1969. IUDs limited. As of 1974, contraceptive instruction required before issuance of marriage license.
1970	1,400	5.2	1950 1960 1970	111 55 33	1963-64	2.3	Official family planning widely available. Also pills and IUDs since late 1960s.

Appendix Table
Selected Demographic, Social, and Economic Characteristics for Selected Developed and Developing Countries, with or without Legal Abortion, Selected Years, 1950-72 (continued)

Developed Countries with Legal Abortion (Year Legalized)	Births per 1,000 Population		Women as % of Total Labor Force		% of All Women in Labor Force		% of Women Aged 15-49 in Labor Force		% of Eligible Women in Secondary School		% Urban of Total Population	
	Year	Rate	Year	%	Year	%	Year	%	Year	%	Year	%
Romania (1956, restricted 1966)	1950-54	24.9	1955	28[a]					1960	37	1950	25
	1960	19.1	1960	28					1965	41	1960	32
	1971	19.6	1967	31	1966	53	1966	73	1969	53	1970	41
Yugoslavia	1950-54	28.8	1956	25					1960	27		
	1960	23.5			1961	31	1961	51	1965	39	1961	28
	1972	18.2	1968	30	1971	31			1969	41	1970	37
U.S.S.R. (1920-36, 1955)	1950-54	26.4										
	1960	24.9	1964	49	1959	49	1959	66[b]	1966	71	1962	51
	1971	17.8			1970	44					1970	56
Japan (1948)	1945-49	30.2	1950	39					1960	77		
	1960	17.2	1960	39					1965	83	1965	68
	1971	19.3	1969	39	1971	38	1971	54	1969	87	1970	72
Scandinavia												
Denmark (1937)	1950-54	17.9	1950	34	1960	28	1960	45	1960	44		
	1960	16.6	1960	31	1965	32	1965	51	1965	36	1962	47
	1971	15.2	1965	30	1971	38			1969	49	1969	45
Sweden (1938)	1950-54	15.5	1950	26					1960	83		
	1960	13.7	1960	30					1965	93	1965	77
	1972	13.8	1965	34	1965	30	1965	47	1969	105	1970	81

[a]Women as percent of total employment in the socialized nonagricultural branches.
[b]Aged 20-59
[c]Urban
[d]Rural

GNP Per Capital in US $		Average Annual Growth Rate of Per Capita GNP	Infant Deaths Per 1,000 Live Births		Average Ideal/ Desired Family Size		Status of Organized Family Planning or Availability of Pill and IUD
Year	Amount	1960-70 %	Year	Rate	Year	Av.	Comment
1970	930	7.7	1964 1970	52 50	1968	2.1[c]	No official family planning. Official importation of pills and IUDs discontinued since 1966.
1970	650	4.3	1964 1971	76 49	1970	2.3-3.8	Organized family planning widespread. Pills available on prescription since late 1960s. IUDs limited.
1960 1970	1,160 2,000	5.8	1964 1970	29 24	1966 1966 1969	1.7[c] 2.8[d] 2.9	Contraceptive advice available. Pills and IUDs restricted.
1950 1960 1970	380 750 1,920	9.6	1964 1970	20 13	1961	2.8	IUDs officially discouraged. High quality condoms widely used. Pills available for menstrual regulation.
1965 1970	1,740 3,190	3.7	1950 1960 1965-70	29 22 15			Organized family planning since 1930s. Pill and IUDs widely available.
1965 1970	2,130 4,040	3.8	1964 1970	14 13	1967	2.4	Organized family planning limited but pills and IUDs available since mid-1960s. Condoms widely advertised.

Appendix Table
Selected Demographic, Social, and Economic Characteristics for Selected Developed and Developing Countries, with or without Legal Abortion, Selected Years, 1950-72 (continued)

Developed Countries with Legal Abortion (Year Legalized)	Births per 1,000 Population		Women as % of Total Labor Force		% of all Women in Labor Force		% of Women Aged 15-49 in Labor Force		% of Eligible Women in Secondary School		% Urban of Total Population	
	Year	Rate	Year	%	Year	%	Year	%	Year	%	Year	%
United States (1967 in some states, 1973 nationally)	1950-54	24.5	1950	28	1950	29[a]	1950	33[b]				
	1960	23.7	1960	32	1960	35[a]	1960	37[b]			1960	70
	1972	15.6	1970	37	1971	43[a]	1970	43[b]	1968	100	1970	74
United Kingdom (1967 in Great Britain)[c]	1950-54	15.9	1951	31					1960	66[d]		
	1960	17.5	1966	37	1966	33			1965	65[d]	1962	80[d]
	1972	14.9			1970	32			1969	72[d]	1971	78[d]
Developed Countries with Restrictive Abortion												
Belgium	1950	16.9							1960	69		
	1960	16.9	1961	27	1961	20	1961	35	1965	62	1962	86
	1972	14.5	1968	31	1971	26					1968	87
France	1950-54	19.5	1954	34					1960	49		
	1960	17.9	1962	35	1962	28	1962	44	1965	59	1962	63
	1972	16.9	1968	35	1968	28	1968	45	1969	74	1968	70
					1972	30						
Greece	1950-54	19.5	1951	18					1960	30		
	1960	16.5	1961	33	1961	28	1961	42	1965	44	1961	44
	1971	16.2			1971	21	1971	32	1969	52		
Italy	1950-54	18.3	1951	26					1960	29		
	1960	18.3	1961	25	1961	20	1961	31	1965	42	1961	48
	1971	16.8	1968	27					1969	51	1970	53

[a] Aged 14 or over

[b] Aged 14-44

GNP Per Capita in US $ Year	GNP Per Capita in US $ Amount	Average Annual Growth Rate of Per Capita GNP 1960-70 %	Infant Deaths Per 1,000 Live Births Year	Infant Deaths Per 1,000 Live Births Rate	Average Ideal/Desired Family Size Year	Average Ideal/Desired Family Size Av	Status of Organized Family Planning or Availability of Pill and IUD Comment
1950	3,515		1950	29	1960	3.1	Pills widely available since early 1960s, IUDs since mid-1960s.
1960	3,710		1960	26	1965	3.3	
1970	4,760	3.2	1970-71	19	1970	2.7	
1950	1,630				1946	2.1[d]	Official family planning 1967. Pills available since early 1960s, IUDs since mid-1960s.
1960	1,855		1960	23	1960	2.8[d]	
1970	2,270	2.2	1972	17[d]	1967	3.4[d]	
					1969	2.9[d]	
			1964	25			Pills and IUDs technically restricted, though available in practice.
1970	2,720	4.0	1970	22	1969	2.7	
1950	1,390				1956	2.2	Pill and IUD import and sales officially restricted but increasingly available from late 1960s.
1960	2,440		1964	23	1960	2.8	
1970	3,100	4.6	1966-70	20	1969	2.7	
			1964	36			IUDs limited. Pills technically restricted but available from mid-1960s.
1970	1,090	6.6	1971	27			
1950	660						Pill available but very limited.
1960	1,100		1964	36	1960	3.1	
1970	1,760	4.6	1970	29	1969	2.6	

[c]United Kingdom includes England and Wales, Scotland, and Northern Ireland. The 1967 Abortion Act applies to Great Britain alone, excluding Northern Ireland. However, pertinent data are seldom available for Great Britain as an entity. Therefore, all data listed here apply to the United Kingdom, except where otherwise indicated.

[d]England and Wales

Appendix Table
Selected Demographic, Social, and Economic Characteristics for Selected Developed and Developing Countries, with or without Legal Abortion, Selected Years, 1950-72 (continued)

Developed Countries with Restrictive Abortion	Births per 1,000 Population		Women as % of Total Labor Force		% of All Women in Labor Force		% of Women Aged 15-49 in Labor Force		% of Eligible Women in Secondary School		% Urban of Total Population	
	Year	Rate	Year	%	Year	%	Year	%	Year	%	Year	%
Netherlands	1950-54	22.1	1956	21					1960	66		
	1960	20.8	1960	22	1960	16	1960	30	1965	63	1962	76
	1972	16.1							1969	66	1970	78
Switzerland	1950-54	17.3	1950	30								
	1960	17.6	1960	30	1960	27	1960	47			1960	51
	1971	15.1	1965	29	1970	32	1970	52	1969	50	1970	55
Developing Countries with Legal or Easily Available Abortion (Year legalized)												
Singapore			1957	18	1957	13			1960	26		
(1970)	1960	38.7							1965	45		
	1972	23.0							1970	51	1971	100
Israel									1960	48		
			1960	26	1961	18	1961	31	1965	51		
	1971	28.5	1968	29	1971	21			1969	60	1970	90
Republic of			1955	47					1960	14	1960	28
Korea	1960	42.9			1966	19	1966	34	1965	25	1966	34
(1973)	1970	29-31	1968	36					1971	38	1970	43
Taiwan	1950	45.9	1950	27							1950	54
	1960	39.5	1960	22	1956	13					1960	58
	1972	24.5	1965	21	1965	13			1970	49	1970	63
Tunisia												
(1965,	1960	48.3			1966	3	1966	6			1966	40
1973)	1968	43.0							1968	11		

[a]Jewish urban

GNP Per Capita in US $		Average Annual Growth Rate of Per Capita GNP	Infant Deaths Per 1,000 Live Births		Average Ideal/ Desired Family Size		Status of Organized Family Planning or Availability of Pill and IUD
Year	Amount	1960-70 %	Year	Rate	Year	Av.	Comment
1950	1,180						Pills available since 1964. IUDs increasing.
1960	1,675		1964	15			
1970	2,430	3.9	1970	12			
			1950	30			Availability of pills and IUDs varies in different cantons.
			1960	21	1960	2.9	
1970	3,320	2.5	1972	14			
			1950	75			Comprehensive official family planning since 1966, with all methods available.
			1960	35			
1970	920	5.2	1970	20			
1950	750		1964	28			No organized family planning. Pills and IUDs available but restricted.
1960	1,200		1967	26			
1970	1,960	4.7	1970	23	1971	3.3[a]	
1950	100				1965	3.9	National program stressing IUDs since 1962. Pills introduced 1968.
1960	135		1966	54	1968	3.9	
1970	250	6.8	1971	46	1971	3.7	
			1950	35	1965	4.0	National program stressing IUDs since 1964. Pills introduced 1967.
1958	124		1960	31	1967	3.8	
1970	390	7.1	1971	19	1970	3.8	
							National program since 1966.
1964	180						
1970	250	0.5	1971	76	1964	4.3	

Appendix Table
Selected Demographic, Social, and Economic Characteristics for Selected Developed and Developing Countries, with or without Legal Abortion, Selected Years, 1950-72 (continued)

Developing Countries with Restrictive Abortion	Births per 1,000 Population		Women as % of Total Labor Force		% of All Women in Labor Force		% of Women Aged 15-49 in Labor Force		% of Eligible Women in Secondary School		% Urban of Total Population	
	Year	Rate	Year	%	Year	%	Year	%	Year	%	Year	%
Albania	1950-54	38.9	1955	42					1960	11		
	1960	43.4	1960	39	1960	36			1965	25	1962	32
	1969	35.3							1969	24	1969	34
Argentina	1952	24.9							1960	32		
	1960	22.5	1960	22	1960	16	1960	28	1965	41	1960	74
	1972	22.0			1970	23			1969	46	1970	80
Brazil	1950	43	1950	15					1960	10		
	1960-66	41-43	1960	18	1960	12	1960	20	1965	17	1960	47
	1965-70	37.8			1970	13	1970	23	1969	25	1970	56
Chile	1950-54	34.3	1952	25					1960	25		
	1960-64	34-36	1960	22	1960	14	1960	25	1965	35	1960	69
	1970	29.6			1971	15			1969	36	1970	76
Colombia			1951	19					1960	11		
	1960-64	41-44	1964	20	1964	12	1964	22	1965	16	1960	48
	1968	44.6							1969	21	1970	60
Mexico			1950	14					1960	6		
	1960-65	44-45	1960	18	1960	12	1960	18	1965	12	1962	53
	1972	43.4	1968	19	1970	10	1970	19	1969	18	1970	59

[a]Urban

GNP Per Capita in US $		Average Annual Growth Rate of Per Capita GNP	Infant Deaths Per 1,000 Live Births		Average Ideal/ Desired Family Size		Status of Organized Family Planning or Availability of Pill and IUD
Year	Amount	1960-70 %	Year	Rate	Year	Av.	Comment
1970	600	4.8	1965	87			No organized family planning, and no importation of pills and IUDs.
1950 1960 1970	785 910 1,160	2.5	1950 1960 1970	65 61 58	1964	2.9[a]	Pill manufacture and import restricted but available.
1950 1960 1970	215 310 420	2.4	1970	88	1964	2.7[a]	Some private clinics since 1965. Pill manufacture and import officially prohibited but available.
1950 1960 1970	560 605 720	1.6	1950 1960 1970	140 128 79	1959	4.1[a]	Organized family planning since 1964. Official support since 1966.
1950 1960 1970	250 290 340	1.7	1950-54 1960 1970	113 100 76	1964 1965	3.6[a] 2.7-5.6	Urban organized family planning since 1965. Pills and IUDs increasingly available since late 1960s.
1950 1960 1970	380 475 670	3.7	1950 1960 1970	96 74 67	1964	4.2[a]	Some private clinics since 1966. Official government support 1973.

Appendix Table
Selected Demographic, Social, and Economic Characteristics for Selected Developed and Developing Countries, with or without Legal Abortion, Selected Years, 1950-72 (continued)

Developing Countries with Restrictive Abortion	Births per 1,000 Population		Women as % of Total Labor Force		% of All Women in Labor Force		% of Women Aged 15-49 in Labor Force		% of Eligible Women in Secondary School		% Urban of Total Population	
	Year	Rate	Year	%	Year	%	Year	%	Year	%	Year	%
Panama			1950	20					1960	31	1962	43
	1960-65	41-42	1960	21	1960	15	1960	27	1965	38	1966	46
	1972	35.6			1970	18	1970	34	1969	42	1971	48
Paraguay			1950	23					1960	5		
	1955-64	42-45	1962	23	1962	14	1962	26	1965	13	1962	36
	1971	44.6							1969	15	1970	36
Peru												
	1960-64	44-45			1961	14	1961	24	1965	23	1966	50
	1968	41.8							1968	32	1971	54
Uruguay									1960	31		
	1960-63	24-25	1963	25	1963	19	1963	33	1965	47	1960	72
	1971	22.6	1970	31					1968	60	1970	78
Venezuela			1950	18					1960	21		
	1960-65	46-48	1961	18	1961	11	1963	22	1965	29	1961	67
	1972	40.9	1971	13					1969	37	1970	76

[a]Urban
[b]Rural
Sources:

Inspiration for this table and guidance to original sources for many of the data presented came from comparable tables appearing in the five editions (to date) of D. Nortman. Population and family planning programs: A factbook. *Reports on Population/Family Planning*, December 1969, July 1970, June 1971, September 1972, September 1973.

Demographic data (crude birth rates, percent urban of total population, infant mortality rates): L.-J.Cho. The demographic situation in the Republic of Korea. Paper presented at the Population Association of America Meeting, New Orleans, Louisiana, April 1973, table 3 (infant mortality rates in Republic of Korea); International Planned Parenthood Federation, *Situation Reports*, various countries, most recent issues; E. Szabady. Interdependence between changes in fertility and the socio-economic development of Eastern European countries, unpublished paper, Budapest: Demographic Institute of the Hungarian Central Statistical Office, 1972, table 2, p. 6 (percent urban of total population in Eastern Europe); United Nations, *Demographic yearbooks*, New York: United Nations, various years; United Nations, Statistical Office, *Population and vital statistics report: Data available as of 1 October 1973*, New York: Author, Statistical Papers, Series A, Vol. 25, Nos. 3 and 4, 1973.

GNP Per Capita in US $		Average Annual Growth Rate of Per Capita GNP	Infant Deaths Per 1,000 Live Births		Average Ideal/ Desired Family Size		Status of Organized Family Planning or Availability of Pill and IUD
Year	Amount	1960-70 %	Year	Rate	Year	Av.	Comment
			1960-65	41	1964	4.2[a]	Private family planning since 1965. Government support 1969.
1970	730	4.2	1970	39			
			1962	98			Limited urban organized family planning since 1969.
1970	260	1.3	1970	84			
			1960-65	62	1960-61	4.0-4.7[a]	Some private urban clinics since 1967. Some commercial sale of pills.
1970	450	1.4	1969	110		5.1[b]	
1950	775						Some private planning since 1963, mainly IUDs.
1960	825		1967	50			
1970	820	−0.4	1970	49			
1950	500		1950	81			Some private family planning services in urban areas, with some government support since 1972.
1960	780		1960	53	1964	3.5[a]	
1970	980	2.3	1971	50			

Women as percent of total employment in the socialized nonagricultural branches, Bulgaria, Czechoslovakia, German Democratic Republic, Hungary, Poland, Romania: A. Elias. Magnitude and distribution of the labor force in Eastern Europe, in United States Congress, Joint Economic Committee, *Economic developments in countries of Eastern Europe: A compendium of papers*, Washington: U.S. Government Printing Office, 1970, table 16, p. 198.

Women as percent of total labor force, other countries various years. Derived from United Nations, Statistical Office, *Demographic yearbook 1970*, New York: Author, 1971, table 12.

Percent of all women in labor force, and *percent of all women aged 15-49 in labor force:* derived from International Labor Organization, *Yearbooks of labor statistics 1968 and 1971*, Geneva: International Labor Organization, 1969, 1972, table 1. United States Department of Commerce, Bureau of the Census, *1970 census of population: General economic and social characteristics, U.S. summary*, Washington: U.S. Government Printing Office, 1972, PC(1)-C1.

Percent of eligible women enrolled in secondary school: UNESCO, *Statistical yearbook 1971*, Paris: Author, 1972, table 2.7.

Gross national product per capita in US $ and *Average annual growth rate of per capita GNP, 1960-70:* World Bank, *World Bank Atlas: Population, per capita product and growth rates*, Washington: World Bank, 1972; World Bank, *Trends in developing countries*, Washington: Author, 1973, tables 2.5 and 2.7.

Average ideal/desired family size: (for Eastern Europe) J. Berent. Causes of fertility decline in Eastern Europe and the Soviet Union–Part III, Family planning and population policies, *Population Studies*, 1970, 24, table 10, p. 283; (USSR 1969) D. Heer. Recent developments in Soviet population policy, *Studies in Family Planning*, 1972, 3, table 3, p. 260; (Yugoslavia 1970) G. Todorovic. Ideal and desired family size, *Stanovnistvo*, 1971, 9, 310-11; (Japan and Western Europe prior to 1965) W.P. Mauldin. Fertility studies in knowledge, attitudes and practices, *Studies in Family Planning*, No. 7, June 1965, pp. 1-10; (Great Britain 1967) M. Woolf. *Family intentions: An enquiry undertaken for the General Registrar's Office*, London: Office of Population Censuses and Surveys, Her Majesty's Stationery Office, 1971, p. 13; (Belgium, France, Great Britain, Italy, 1969) International Health Foundation, *Family planning: A study of the attitudes, knowledge, and practice of women in Italy, Belgium, France, Great Britain, and West Germany, 1969*, Geneva: Author, 1971, p. 6.; (Israel) D. Friedlander. Family planning in Israel: Irrationality and ignorance, *Journal of Marriage and the Family*, 1973, 35, table 1, p. 119; (Latin America) H. Mendoza-Hoyos. Research studies on abortion and family planning in Colombia, *Milbank Memorial Fund Quarterly*, 1968, Part 2, 36, table 9, p. 230; C. Miro. Some misconceptions disproved: A program of comparative fertility studies in Latin America, in B. Berelson et al. (eds.), *Family planning and population programs*, Chicago: University of Chicago Press, 1966, table 16, p. 632; J.M. Stycos. Social class and preferred family size in Peru, in J.M. Stycos (ed.), *Human fertility in Latin America*, Ithaca, N.Y.: Cornell University Press, 1968; (Republic of Korea) H.-S.Moon, S.-H. Han, and S. Choi. *Fertility and family planning: An interim report on 1971 fertility-abortion survey*, Seoul: Korean Institute for Family Planning, February 1973, table III-10, p. 78; (Sweden) G. Svala. Sweden, *Country Profiles*, July 1972, p. 13; (Taiwan) R. Freedman, L.C. Coombs, and M.-C. Chang. Trends in family-size preferences and practice of family planning: Taiwan, 1965-1970, *Studies in Family Planning*, 1972, 3, table 4, p. 284; (Tunisia) D.J. Bogue. *Principles of demography*, New York: Wiley, 1969, table 20-3, p. 843; (United States) F.S. Jaffe. Family planning services in the United States, in R. Parke, Jr., and C.F. Westoff (eds.), *Aspects of population growth policy.* Vol. 6 of the Commission on Population Growth and the American Future Research Reports, Washington: U.S. Government Printing Office, 1972, table 1, p. 207, and table 8, p. 213.

Family planning/contraceptive information: H.P. David. *Family planning and abortion in the socialist countries of Central and Eastern Europe*, New York: The Population Council, 1970; International Planned Parenthood Federation, *Family planning in five continents*, London, October 1973; International Planned Parenthood Federation, *Situation Reports*, various countries, most recent issues; D. Nortman. Population and family planning programs: A factbook, *Reports on Population/Family Planning*, September 1973, table 6.

References

References

1. Abernathy, J.R., Greenberg, B.G., and Horvitz, D.G. Estimates of induced abortion in urban North Carolina. *Demography*, 1970, 7, 19-29.
2. Acsadi, G., Klinger, A., and Szabady, E. *Studies on family planning–II: Main results of the 1966 fertility and family planning study (TCS-66)*. Budapest: Demographic Research Institute of the Hungarian Central Statistical Office and the Committee for Demography of the Hungarian Academy of Sciences, 1970.
3. af Geijerstam, G. Abortion in Scandinavia. In R.E. Hall (ed.), *Abortion in a changing world.* Vol. 1. New York: Columbia University Press, 1970, pp. 315-24.
4. Agualimpia, C., Mejía, A., and Paredes, R., et al. *Investigación nacional de morbilidad, los hechos demográficos.* Bogota: Public Health Ministry and Colombian Association of Faculties of Medicine, 1968.
5. Aguirre, Z.F.J., Ramírez, S.E., and León, M.C. Epidemiología del aborto ilegal. Paper presented to the Vth Congress of Gynecology and Obstetrics, Mexico City, June 1967.
6. Aird, J.S. Population policy and demographic prospects in the People's Republic of China. In United States Congress, Joint Economic Committee of, People's Republic of China: An economic assessment. Washington: U.S. Government Printing Office, 1972, pp. 220-31.
7. Alpana, A. El aborto provocado como problema de salud pública. Paper presented at the XVIth Annual Meeting of the Mexican Association of Hygiene, Mexico City, 1962.
8. American Law Institute. *Abortion: Model Penal Code.* Philadelphia: Author, 1962.
9. *American Medical Association Gazette.* March 13, 1973.
10. Armijo, R., and Monreal, T. Epidemiology of provoked abortion in Santiago, Chile. *The Journal of Sex Research*, 1965, 1, 143-59.
11. Armijo, R., and Monreal, T. The problem of induced abortion in Chile. *Milbank Memorial Fund Quarterly*, 1965, 43(4), 263-80.
12. Aso, T. Fertility control transition from abortion to contraceptives in Japan since 1948. Paper prepared for Population Association of America Meeting, Toronto, April 1972.
13. Bachi, R. Abortion in Israel. In R.E. Hall (ed.), *Abortion in a changing world.* Vol. 1. New York: Columbia University Press, 1970, pp. 274-83.
14. Bauman, K.E., and Udry, J.R. The difference in unwanted births between blacks and whites. *Demography*, 1973, 10, 315-28.
15. Berelson, B. The present state of family planning programs. *Studies in Family Planning*, September 1970, No. 57, pp. 1-11.
16. Berelson, B. An evaluation of the effects of population control programs. Unpublished paper delivered at Oxford University, March 1973.

17. Berent, J. Causes of fertility decline in Eastern Europe and the Soviet Union—Part I: The influence of demographic factors; Part II: Economic and social factors; Part III: Family planning and population policies. *Population Studies*, 1970, 24, 35-58, 247-92.
18. Berent, J., and Festy, P. Measuring the impact of some demographic factors on postwar trends in crude birth rates in Europe. In International Union for the Scientific Study of Population, *International Population Conference, Liège, 1973.* Vol. 2 Liège: Author, 1973, pp. 99-112.
19. Berkov, B., and Sklar, J. *The impact of legalized abortion on fertility in California.* Berkeley: University of California, International Population and Urban Research, Results of Current Research in Demography, Preliminary Paper No. 1, 1972.
20. Birmingham Pregnancy Advisory Service. *Provision for abortion: Whose responsibility?* Author's memorandum submitted to the Official Committee on the Working of the Abortion Act, United Kingdom, December 1971.
21. Bogue, D.J. *Principles of demography.* New York: Wiley, 1969.
22. Bone, M. *Family planning services in England and Wales: An enquiry carried out on behalf of the Department of Health and Social Security, Office of Population Censuses and Surveys.* London: Her Majesty's Stationery Office, 1973.
23. Borell, U., and Engstrom, L. Legal abortions in Sweden. *World Medical Journal*, 1966, 13(3), 72-75.
24. Braestrup, A. Use of contraception by young mothers in Copenhagen. *Journal of Biosocial Science*, 1971, 3, 43-60.
25. Breznik, D. The survey of fertility of married women and family planning. (English summary) *Stanovnistvo*, 1971, 9, 202-205.
26. Brudenell, M. Foreword to A. Hordern, *Legal abortion: The English experience*. Oxford: Pergamon Press, 1971.
27. Bulgaria, Government of. Law on interruption of pregnancy. *International Digest of Health Legislation*, 1957, 8, 605-607.
28. Bulgaria, Ministry of National Health. *Instruction No. 188*, January 1968, amended by Instructions 0-10 and 0-27 of May 1972 and April 1973, respectively.
29. Bumpass, L.L., and Presser, H.B. The increasing acceptance of sterilization and abortion. In C.F. Westoff et al., *Towards the end of growth: Population in America.* Englewood Cliffs, N.J.: Prentice-Hall, 1973, pp. 33-46.
30. Burnhill, M.S. The effect of different induced abortion policies on maternal health, birth rate and natural increase. Unpublished paper, State University of New York, Department of Obstetrics and Gynecology, 1971.
31. Calderone, M.S. *Abortion in the United States.* New York: Hoeber-Harper, 1958.
32. California, Senate of. An act to add Chapter 11 to Division 20 of the Health

and Safety Code, to amend Section 2377 of the Business and Professions Code, and to amend Sections 274, 275, and 276 of the Penal Code relating to abortion. *Senate Bill No. 462*, amended May 1, 1967.

33. Callahan, D. *Abortion: Law, choice and morality.* New York: Macmillan, 1970.
34. Campbell, A. Role of family planning in reduction of poverty. *Journal of Marriage and the Family*, 1968, 30, 236-45.
35. Campbell, A. Three generations of parents. *Family Planning Perspectives*, 1973, 5, 106-12.
36. Carrasco, E. Incidence of abortion, fertility and contraception in Latin America. In International Union for the Scientific Study of Population, *International Population Conference, Liège, 1973.* Vol. 2. Liège: Author, 1973, pp. 297-314.
37. Cartwright, A. England and Wales: General practitioners and family planning. *Studies in Family Planning*, July 1968, No. 32, pp. 10-15.
38. Cartwright, A., and Waite, M. General practitioners and abortion: Evidence to the Committee on the Working of the Abortion Act. *Journal of Royal College of General Practitioners*, 1972, 22 (Supplement 1), 1-24.
39. Chang, K.S., Worth, G.C., Watson, W.B., and Michael, P.H. Korea (South). *Studies in Family Planning*, 1973, 4, 107-11.
40. Chen, P.-c. China's population program at the grass-roots level. *Studies in Family Planning* 1973, 4, 219-27.
41. Cho, L.-J. Economic and demographic influences on the family in Korea. In National Institutes of Health, Fogarty International Center, *The family in transition: A round table conference*, Bethesda, Maryland, November 1969. Washington; U.S. Government Printing Office, Fogarty International Center Proceedings No. 3, 1971, pp. 139-54.
42. Cho, L.-J. The demographic situation in the Republic of Korea. Paper presented at the Population Association of America Meeting, New Orleans, Louisiana, April 1973.
43. Cho, L.-J., and Retherford, R.D. Comparative analysis of recent fertility trends in East Asia. In International Union for the Scientific Study of Population, *International Population Conference, Liège, 1973.* Vol. 2. Liège: Author, 1973, pp. 163-81.
44. Chow, L.P. Abortion in Taiwan. In R.E. Hall (ed.), *Abortion in a changing world.* Vol. 1. New York: Columbia University Press, 1970, pp. 251-59.
45. Chow, L.P. Measurement of the incidence of abortion: Preliminary results from a study in Taiwan. Paper presented at the International Union for the Scientific Study of Population, Workshop on Abortion, University of North Carolina, Chapel Hill, March 1973.
46. Chow, L.P., et al. The impact of reform of abortion laws in Taiwan. Study in progress based in part on findings from the epidemiological study on the outcome of pregnancy conducted by School of Hygiene and Public Health,

The Johns Hopkins University, Baltimore, Maryland. Personal communication, July 1973.

47. Conning, A.M. Latin American fertility trends and influencing factors. In International Union for the Scientific Study of Population, *International Population Conference, Liège, 1973.* Vol. 2. Liège: Author, 1973, pp. 125-48.
48. Cossey, D. Free contraception and the NHS Reorganization Bill. *Family Planning*, 1973, 22, 53-54.
49. Cutright, P. Illegitimacy in the United States: 1920-1968. In C.F. Westoff and R. Parke, Jr. (eds.), *Demographic and social aspects of population growth.* Vol. 1 of the Commission on Population Growth and the American Future Research Reports. Washington: U.S. Government Printing Office, 1972, pp. 375-438.
50. Cutright, P., and Galle, O. The effect of illegitimacy on U.S. general fertility rates and population growth. *Population Studies*, 1973, 27, 515-26.
51. Czechoslovakia, Government of. Law on interruption of pregnancy. *International Digest of Health Legislation*, 1959, 10, 283-92.
52. Czechoslovakia, Government of. Decree No. 54 of 6 July 1966. *International Digest of Health Legislation*, 1968, 19, 173-75.
53. Czechoslovakia, Government of. Ordinance of the Government of the Czech Socialist Republic of 16 May 1973 to repeal in part Government Ordinance No. 126/1962 to establish committees for the interruption of pregnancy and applying the law on the artificial interruption of pregnancy. (In Czech) *Sbirka Zakonu*, 1973, Castka 20, various pages.
54. David, H.P. *Family planning and abortion in the socialist countries of Central and Eastern Europe.* New York: The Population Council, 1970.
55. David, H.P. Observations on family planning and abortion in Sweden: Notes on a March 1972 visit to Stockholm. Washington: AIR/Transnational Family Research Institute, Memorandum, 1972.
56. David, H.P. Abortion and family planning in the Soviet Union: Public policies and private behaviors. Paper presented at the Symposium on "The Soviet Population Crisis," Ohio State University, Columbus, April 1973.
57. David, H.P., Alam, Z., and Kalis, M.G. *Abortion legislation: A summary international classification.* Washington: AIR/Transnational Family Research Institute, 1972 (updated to March 1974).
58. David, H.P., Kalis, M.G., and Tietze, C. *Selected abortion statistics: An international summary.* Washington: AIR/Transnational Family Research Institute, 1973 (updated to March 1974).
59. David, H.P., and Russo, N.F. Abortion and fertility regulation in the socialist countries of Central and Eastern Europe. In S.H. Newman, M.B. Beck, and S. Lewit (eds.), *Abortion, obtained and denied: Research approaches.* New York: The Population Council, 1971, pp. 81-96.
60. David, H.P., and Wright, N.H. Abortion legislation: The Romanian experience. *Studies in Family Planning*, 1971, 2, 205-10.

61. Davis, K. The theory of change and response in modern demographic history. *Population Index*, 1963, 29, 345-66.
62. Denmark, Government of. Law No. 177 of 23 June 1956 on measures to be taken in cases of pregnancy, etc. *International Digest of Health Legislation*, 1957, 8, 377-81.
63. Denmark, Government of. Law No. 120 of 24 March 1970. *International Digest of Health Legislation*, 1970, 21, 572-76.
64. Denmark, Government of. Law No. 350 of 13 June 1973 on the interruption of pregnancy. *Lovtidende for Kongeriget Danmark*, Part A, 6 July 1973, No. 32, pp. 993-95.
65. Diggory, P. Some experience of therapeutic abortion. *The Lancet*, 1969, 1, 873.
66. Diggory, P. The unwanted pregnancy. *Journal of Biosocial Science*, 1971 (Supplement 3), pp. 127-32.
67. Diggory, P., Peel, J., and Potts, M. Preliminary assessment of the 1967 abortion act in practice. *The Lancet*, 1970, 1, 287-91.
68. District of Columbia, Department of Human Resources. *Therapeutic abortions in the District of Columbia, 1972.* Washington: Author, 1973.
69. Dixon, R.B. Explaining cross-cultural variations in age at marriage and proportions never-marrying. *Population Studies*, 1971, 25, 215-32.
70. Erhardt, C., Tietze, C., and Nelson, F. United States: Therapeutic abortions in New York City. *Studies in Family Planning*, 1970, No. 51, pp. 8-9.
71. Fabery, I. *Abortion and birth-rate in the Netherlands: Summary of a report made for the State Committee for Population Problems.* Zeist: Dutch Institute for Social Sexological Research, 1973.
72. Faundes, A., and Luukkainen, T. Health and family planning services in the Chinese People's Republic. *Studies in Family Planning*, 1972, 3(7) (Supplement), 165-76.
73. Faundes, A., Rodriguez-Galant, G., and Avendano, O. The San Gregorio experimental family planning program: Changes observed in fertility and abortion rates. *Demography*, 1968, 5, 836-45.
74. Fessler, L. Delayed marriage and planned birth. *Fieldstaff Reports*, East Asia Series, 1973, 20(1), 1-15.
75. Field, M.G. The re-legalization of abortion in Soviet Russia. *New England Journal of Medicine*, 1956, 255, 421-27.
76. Figa-Talamanca, I. The relationship of contraception to abortion in Japan. *Genus*, 1970, 26, 237-58.
77. Finland, Government of. Law No. 82 of 17 February 1950 relating to the interruption of pregnancy. *International Digest of Health Legislation*, 1951, 2, 559-61.
78. Finland, Government of. Law No. 239 of 24 March 1970. *International Digest of Health Legislation*, 1970, 21, 699-705.
79. Frederiksen, H., and Brackett, J.W. Demographic effects of abortion. *Public Health Reports*, 1968, 83, 999-1010.

80. Freedman, R., Coombs, L.C., and Chang, M.-C. Trends in family-size preferences and practice of family planning: Taiwan, 1965-1970. *Studies in Family Planning*, 1972, 3, 281-96.

81. Freedman, R., Hermalin, A., and Sun, T. Fertility trends in Taiwan, 1961-1970. *Population Index*, 1972, 38, 141-66.

82. Friedlander, D. Family planning in Israel: Irrationality and ignorance. *Journal of Marriage and the Family*, 1973, 35, 117-24.

83. Friedlander, D., and Sabatello, E. Israel. *Country Profiles*, February 1972.

84. Gall, N. Births, abortions and the progress of Chile. *Fieldstaff Reports*, West Coast South America Series, 1972, 19(2), 1-10.

85. Gaslonde, S. Abortion-fertility studies in Asuncion, Bogota, Buenos Aires, Lima, and Panama. In H.P. David and S. Cambiaso (eds.), *Abortion and family planning practices in Latin America.* Washington: Pan American Health Organization, 1974, forthcoming.

86. Gaslonde, S., and Carrasco, E. *A survey to evaluate the efficacy of the family planning programs: With application to five cities in Paraguay.* (In Spanish) Santiago: Centro Latino Americano de Demografia (CELADE), 1973, Series A, No. 119.

87. Goode, W.J. *World revolution and family patterns.* London: Free Press of Glencoe, 1963.

88. Goodhart, C.B. The frequency of illegal abortion. *Eugenics Review*, 1964, 55, 197-200.

89. Goodhart, C.B. On the incidence of illegal abortion. *Population Studies*, 1973, 27, 207-34.

90. Gutiérrez, H. Algunas consideraciones sobre el nivel de abortos in Costa Rica en el año 1963. Unpublished paper, University of California, International Population and Urban Research, July 1966.

91. Han, D.W. The Republic of Korea. *Country Profiles*, April 1970.

92. Han, S.H. *The study on induced abortion: 1971 fertility-abortion survey.* Seoul: Korean Institute for Family Planning, Special Report Series, No. 2, April 1973.

93. Hanna, W.A. Singapore success syndrome retested. *Fieldstaff Reports*, Southeast Asia Series, 1973, 21(3), 1-15.

94. Harris, D., O'Hare, D., Pakter, J., and Nelson, F.G. Legal abortion 1970-71: The New York City experience. *American Journal of Public Health*, 1973, 63, 409-18.

95. Heer, D. The demographic transition in the Russian Empire and the Soviet Union. *Journal of Social History*, Spring 1968, pp. 193-240.

96. Hervet, E. In search of the truth about abortion. (In French) *Gynecologie et Obstetrique et Federation des Sociétés de Gynecologie et d'Obstetrique de la Langue Française*, 1970, 69, 287-95.

97. Hong, S.-B. Induced abortion in rural Korea. *Korean Journal of Obstetrics and Gynecology*, 1967, 10, 275-95.

98. Hong, S.-B. *Changing patterns of induced abortion in Seoul, Korea.* Seoul: The Population Council, 1971.
99. Hong, S.-B. Impact of induced abortion on birth rates in Korea. *Korean Journal of Population Problems*, May 1973.
100. Hubinont, P.O., Brat, T., Polderman, J., and Ramdoyal, R. Abortion in Western Europe. In R.E. Hall (ed.), *Abortion in a changing world.* Vol. 1. New York: Columbia University Press, 1970, pp. 325-37.
101. Hulka, J.F. A mathematical model study of contraceptive efficiency and unplanned pregnancies. *American Journal of Obstetrics and Gynecology*, 1969, 104, 443-47.
102. Hungary, Government of. Order No. 1047/1956 of 3 June 1956 and Ordinance No. 2/1956 of 24 June 1956. *International Digest of Health Legislation*, 1958, 9, 536-40.
103. Hungary, Government of. Decision No. 1040/1973/x.18 of the Council of Ministers on the Tasks of Population Policy. *Magyar Közlöngy*, 1973, No. 71, pp. 777-78.
104. India, Government of, Ministry of Health and Family Planning. *Report of the Committee to Study the Legalization of Abortion.* Delhi: Author, 1966.
105. India, Government of. Medical termination of pregnancy rules, 1973. *International Digest of Health Legislation*, 1972, 23, 771-75.
106. International Health Foundation. *Family planning: A study of the attitudes, knowledge, and practice of women in Italy, Belgium, France, Great Britain, and West Germany*. Geneva: Author, 1971.
107. International Planned Parenthood Federation. *Situation Reports*, various countries, most recent issues.
108. International Planned Parenthood Federation. Improved contraception in Hungary. *IPPF Medical Bulletin*, 1971, 5(4), 3.
109. International Planned Parenthood Federation. *Legal abortions in Britain.* London: Author, 1972.
110. Jaffe, F.S. Family planning services in the United States. In R. Parke, Jr. and C.F. Westoff (eds.), *Aspects of population growth policy*. Vol. 6 of the Commission on Population Growth and the American Future Research Reports. Washington: U.S. Government Printing Office, 1972, pp. 205-52.
111. James, W.H. The incidence of illegal abortion. *Population Studies*, 1971, 25, 327-39.
112. Japan, Government of, Ministry of Health and Welfare. *Yu Sei Ho Go Tokei Ho Koku.* Tokyo: Author, published annually.
113. Japan, Government of. Law No. 156 of 13 July 1948, including amendments up to 21 April 1960. *International Digest of Health Legislation*, 1965, 16, 690.
114. Jarvinen, P.A. Legal abortions in Finland. *Annales Chururgiae et Gynecology Fenniae*, 1971, 60, 65-66.

115. Kanagaratnam, K. Singapore: The national family planning program. *Studies in Family Planning*, 1968, No. 28, pp. 1-15.
116. Kapor-Stanulovic, N., and Beric, B. Family planning in Yugoslavia with special reference to the province of Vojvodina. *Journal of Biosocial Science*, 1973, 5, 179-85.
117. Katagiri, T. A report on the family planning program in the People's Republic of China. *Studies in Family Planning*, 1973, 4, 216-18.
118. Kee, W.F. Singapore. *Studies in Family Planning*, 1972, 3, 143-45.
119. Kee, W.F. Singapore family planning and population board experience with legalized abortion. Paper presented at International Union for the Scientific Study of Population, Workshop on Abortion, University of North Carolina, Chapel Hill, March 1973.
120. Kee, W.F., and Lee, A.S. Singapore. *Studies in Family Planning*, 1973, 4, 117-18.
121. Kind, R.W. Young opinions. *Family Planning*, 1969, 18, 121-24.
122. Klinger, A. Demographic aspects of abortion. In *Conference Proceedings: International Union for the Scientific Study of Population*, London, September 1969. Liège: Author, 1970, pp. K4.21-K4.29.
123. Klinger, A. Longitudinal study of Hungarian women married in 1966. Unpublished paper, Demographic Research Institute of the Hungarian Central Statistical Office, Budapest, 1973.
124. Korea, Republic of. *Maternal and child health, family planning, abortion, and sterilization law.* Seoul: The Population Council, 1973 (unofficial translation).
125. Koya, Y. Why induced abortions in Japan remain high. In Y. Koya (ed.), *Pioneering in family planning: A collection of papers on the family planning programs and research conducted in Japan.* New York: The Population Council, 1963, pp. 76-84.
126. Kwa, S.B., Quah, S.T., and Cheng, M.C.E. The abortion act, 1969: A review of the first year's experience. *Singapore Medical Journal*, 1971, 12, 250-55.
127. Langford, C.M. Birth control practice in Britain. *Family Planning*, 1969, 17, 87-92.
128. Lapham, R.J. Family planning and fertility in Tunisia. *Demography*, 1970, 7, 241-53.
129. Lapham, R.J., and Mauldin, W.P. National family planning programs: Review and evaluation. *Studies in Family Planning*, 1972, 3, 29-52.
130. Lauritsen, J.G., and Haack-Sorenson, P.E. Legal induced abortion: The first year under the new abortion law. (In Danish with English summary) *Ugeskrift Laeger*, 1972, 134, 405-10.
131. Lee, L.T. Five largest countries allow legal abortion on broad grounds. *Population Report*, April 1973, Series F, No. 1.
132. Lee, T.Y. Taiwan. *Studies in Family Planning*, 1972, 3, 145-50.
133. Lewis-Faning, E. *Family limitation and its influence on human fertility.* London: His Majesty's Stationery Office, 1949.

134. Loewenthal, N.H., and David, A.S. *Social and economic correlates of family fertility: An updated review of the evidence.* Research Triangle Park, N.C.: Research Triangle Institute, 1972.

135. Maryland, State of, Department of Health and Mental Hygiene. Article 43, Sections 137-139 of The Health Laws of Maryland, 1970 Cumulative Supplement. Reproduced by Maryland Center for Health Statistics, May 1971.

136. Matsumoto, Y.S., Koizumi, A., and Nohara, T. Condom use in Japan. *Studies in Family Planning*, 1972, 3, 251-55.

137. McDonald, C. Unmet needs in family planning. *People*, 1973, 1(1), 3-6.

138. McIntyre, R.J. The effects of liberalized abortion laws in Eastern Europe. In R.L. Clinton and K. Godwin (eds.), *Research in the politics of population.* Lexington, Mass.: Heath, 1972, pp. 183-216.

139. McIntyre, R.J. The fertility response to abortion reform in Eastern Europe: Demographic and economic implications. *American Economist*, 1972, 16, 45-63.

140. McIntyre, R.J. Pronatalist policies in European socialist countries. Paper presented at International Union for the Scientific Study of Population, Liège, August 1973.

141. Mehlan, K.-H. Legal abortions in Roumania. *Journal of Sex Research*, 1965, 1, 31-38.

142. Miro, C., and Mertens, W. Influences affecting fertility in urban and rural Latin America. *Milbank Memorial Fund Quarterly*, 1968, 46(3), Part 2, 89-117.

143. Monreal, T., and Armijo, R. Evaluation of the programme for the prevention of induced abortion and for family planning in the City of Santiago. *Revista Médica de Chile*, 1968, 96, 605-22.

144. Moon, H.-S., Han, S.-H., and Choi, S. *Fertility and family planning: An interim report on 1971 fertility-abortion survey.* Seoul: Korean Institute for Family Planning, 1973.

145. Moore, E. Induced abortion and contraception: Sociological aspects. In S.H. Newman, M.B. Beck, and S. Lewit (eds.), *Abortion, obtained and denied: Research approaches.* New York: The Population Council, 1971, pp. 131-56.

146. Moore-Cavar, E.C. *Inventory of information on induced abortion.* New York: Columbia University, International Institute for the Study of Human Reproduction, 1974.

147. Muramatsu, M. (ed.). *Japan's experience in family planning–past and present.* Tokyo: Family Planning Federation of Japan, 1967.

148. Muramatsu, M. The demographic aspects of abortion in Japan. In International Planned Parenthood Federation, *Some significant publications on induced abortion.* London: Author, 1971, pp. 84-88.

149. Muramatsu, M. Japan. *Country Profiles*, March 1971.

150. Muramatsu, M. Incidence of abortion in Japan: Analyses and results. In

International Union for the Scientific Study of Population, *International Population Conference, Liège, 1973.* Vol. 2. Liège: Author, 1973, pp. 319-31.

151. Muramatsu, M. The Japanese experience. In H.P. David (ed.), *Abortion research reader.* Lexington, Mass.: Lexington Books, 1974, forthcoming.

152. Myers, P.F. Demographic trends in Eastern Europe. In United States Congress, Joint Economic Committee of, *Economic development in countries of Eastern Europe: A compendium of papers.* Washington: U.S. Government Printing Office, 1970, pp. 68-148.

153. Myrdal, A., and Myrdal, G. *Crisis in the population question.* Stockholm: Bonnier, 1934.

154. New York, State of. *An act to amend the penal law in relation to justifiable abortional acts by physicians in the course of their practice of medicine. Amendment of Section 1, Subdivision 3 of section 125.05 of the penal law, effective July 1, 1970.* Albany: Author, Assembly Print 12,005, 1970.

155. *The New York Times.* The pill works–if you take it. September 23, 1973.

156. Nortman, D. Population and family planning programs: A factbook. *Reports on Population/Family Planning*, December 1969, July 1970, June 1971, September 1972, September 1973.

157. Nortman, D. Status of national family planning programmes of developing countries in relation to demographic targets. *Population Studies*, 1972, 26, 5-13.

158. Norway, Government of. Law No. 2 of 11 November 1960. *International Digest of Health Legislation*, 1965, 16, 148-51.

159. Ohrberg, K. Legal abortion in Sweden. *World Medical Journal*, 1970, 4, 84-86.

160. Omran, A.R. Abortion in the demographic transition. In R. Revelle (ed.), *Rapid population growth: Consequences and policy implications*. Vol. 2. Baltimore: The Johns Hopkins Press, 1971, pp. 479-532.

161. Ottosson, J.O. Legal abortion in Sweden: Thirty years' experience. *Journal of Biosocial Science*, 1971, 3, 173-92.

162. Pakter, J., Harris, D., and Nelson, F. Surveillance of the abortion program in New York City: Preliminary report. *Modern Treatment*, 1971, 8, 169-201.

163. Pakter, J., O'Hare, D., Nelson, F., and Svigir, M. Two years' experience in New York City with the liberalized abortion law: Progress and problems. *American Journal of Public Health*, 1973, 63, 524-35.

164. Pannell, C. Three years' experience of the working of the abortion act in Britain. *New Zealand Medical Journal*, 1972, 76, 117-19.

165. Peel, J. The Hull family survey: II. *Journal of Biosocial Science*, 1972, 4, 333-46.

166. Peel, J. Patterns of fertility. *Journal of Biosocial Science*, 1973, 5, 244-49.

167. Peel, J., and Potts, M. Demographic aspects of abortion in Britain. Paper

presented at the International Union for the Scientific Study of Population Meeting, London, September 1969.

168. Peel, J., and Potts, M. *Textbook of contraceptive practice.* New York: Cambridge University Press, 1969.

169. Planned Parenthood Federation. *The New York abortion story.* New York: Author, 1972.

170. Plaza, S., and Briones, H. El aborto como problema asistencial. *Revista Médica de Chile*, 1963, 91, 294-97.

171. Poland, Government of. Law No. 61 of 27 April 1956. *International Digest of Health Legislation*, 1958, 9, 319-23.

172. The Population Problems Research Council of the Mainichi Newspapers. *Summaries of ninth, tenth, and eleventh national surveys on family planning.* Tokyo: Author, 1968, 1971, 1972.

173. Population Reference Bureau. *World population data sheets.* Washington: Author, various years.

174. Potter, R.E. Additional births averted when abortion is added to contraception. *Studies in Family Planning*, 1972, 3, 53-59.

175. Potts, M. Legal abortion in Eastern Europe. *Eugenics Review*, 1967, 59, 232-50.

176. Potts, M. Abortion and contraception. Lecture delivered at Margaret Pyke House, London, June 1972.

177. Potts, M. Introduction: Problems and strategy. In M. Potts and C. Woods (eds.), *New concepts in contraception.* Baltimore: University Park Press, 1972, pp. 1-16.

178. Potts, M. Models for progress: United Kingdom (1919-1939) and China People's Republic (1957-1971). In M. Potts and C. Woods (eds.), *New concepts in contraception.* Baltimore: University Park Press, 1972, pp. 213-28.

179. Potts, M. Abortion in Western Europe and Africa. Paper presented at International Union for the Scientific Study of Population, Workshop on Abortion, University of North Carolina, Chapel Hill, March 1973.

180. Potts, M. Personal communication, November 6, 1973.

181. Potts, M. The role of family planning in the world population crisis. *Clinics in Endocrinology and Metabolism*, 1973, 2, 577-88.

182. Potts, M., Diggory, P., and Peel, J. *Abortion: A study in medical sociology.* Cambridge, England: Cambridge University Press, 1974, in press.

183. Ravenholt, R.T., Brackett, J.W., and Chao, J. Family planning programs and fertility patterns. *Population Reports*, August 1973, Series J, No. 1.

184. Redford, M.H., and Marcuse, E.K. *Legal abortion in Washington State: An analysis of the first year's experience.* Seattle: Battelle, 1973.

185. Requena, M. Social and economic correlates of induced abortion in Chile. *Demography*, 1965, 2, 33-40.

186. Requena, M. The problem of induced abortion in Latin America. *Demography*, 1968, 5, 785-99.

187. Requena, M. Abortion in Latin America. In R.E. Hall (ed.), *Abortion in a changing world.* Vol. 1. New York: Columbia University Press, 1970, pp. 338-52.

188. Requena, M., and Monreal, T. Evaluation of induced abortion control and family planning programs in Chile. *Milbank Memorial Fund Quarterly*, 1968, 46(3), 191-211.

189. Research Triangle Institute. *Social and economic correlates of family fertility: A survey of the evidence.* Research Triangle Park, N.C.: Author, 1971.

190. Rich, W. *Smaller families through social and economic progress.* Washington: Overseas Development Council, Monograph No. 7, 1973.

191. Romania, Government of. Decree No. 770 of 29 September 1966. *International Digest of Health Legislation*, 1967, 18, 822-37.

192. Romanian Communist Party, Central Committee. Analiza starii de senatate a populatiei si masurile privind perfectionarea organizarii retelei sanitare se imbunatatirea asistentei medicale in Republica Socialista Romania. (In Romanian) *Scinteia*, October 27, 1968.

193. Rosada, I. Situación del aborto voluntario en el Uruguay. Paper presented at International Planned Parenthood Federation Congress, Puerto Rico, 1964.

194. Rosenwaike, I. Therapeutic abortion and fertility in Maryland, 1960-1971. Paper presented at Population Association of America Meeting, New Orleans, Louisiana, April 1973.

195. Ross, J.A., Germain, A., Forrest, J.E., and van Ginneken, J. Findings from family planning research. *Reports on Population/Family Planning*, October 1972, No. 12.

196. Ross, J.A., and Han, D.W. Korea, 1969: Report on the national family planning program. *Studies in Family Planning*, 1970, No. 54, pp. 1-16.

197. Royal College of Obstetricians and Gynaecologists. *Unplanned pregnancy: Report of the working party.* London: Author, 1972.

198. Ryder, N.B. Contraceptive failure in the United States. *Family Planning Perspectives*, 1973, 5, 133-42.

199. Ryder, N.B., and Westoff, C.F. *Reproduction in the United States, 1965.* Princeton, N.J.: Princeton University Press, 1971.

200. Ryder, N.B., and Westoff, C.F. Wanted and unwanted fertility in the United States, 1965-70. In C.F. Westoff and R. Parke, Jr. (eds.), *Demographic and social aspects of population growth.* Vol. 1 of the Commission on Population Growth and the American Future Research Reports. Washington: U.S. Government Printing Office, 1972, pp. 646-58.

201. Salazar, J.H. Aspectos demográficos de la fecundidad en Lima Metropolitana. *Boletín de Análisis Demográfico*, Ministerio de Hacienda y Comercio, Dirección General de Estadística y Censos, 1968, No. 8.

202. Santee, B. A prospective study of abortion in Santiago, Chile. In H.P. David

and S. Cambiaso (eds.), *Abortion and family planning practices in Latin America.* Washington: Pan American Health Organization, 1974, forthcoming.

203. Sarvis, B., and Rodman, H. *The abortion controversy.* New York: Columbia University Press, 1973.
204. Sele, V., and Norgaard, M. Developments in the incidence of abortion in recent years: Investigations and calculations concerning the incidence of criminal abortions prior to and after the Danish abortion law of 1970. (In Danish with English summary) *Ugeskrift for Laeger*, 1972, 134, 2493-505.
205. Simms, M. The abortion act after three years. *Political Quarterly*, 1971, 42, 269-86.
206. Simms, M. Great Britain. In H.P. David (ed.), *Abortion research reader.* Lexington, Mass.: Lexington Books, 1974, forthcoming.
207. Singapore, Government of. The abortion act, 1969 (No. 25 of 1969). In Republic of Singapore, *Government Gazette, Acts Supplement*, January 9, 1970, No. 13, pp. 121-35.
208. Sjovall, H. Abortion and contraception in Sweden, 1870-1970. *Zeitschrift für Rechtsmedizin*, 1972, 70, 197-209.
209. Sklar, J., and Berkov, B. The effects of legal abortion on legitimate and illegitimate birth rates: The California experience. *Studies in Family Planning*, 1973, 4, 281-92.
210. Srb, V. Research in marriage reproduction (1970). *Demosta*, 1972, 5, 442-49.
211. Stamm, H. Abortion situation in Switzerland. (In German with English summary) *Geburtshilfe und Frauenheilkunde*, 1971, 31, 241-50.
212. Stampar, D. Demographic and other effects of the liberalization of abortion legislation in the Republic of Croatia. Paper presented at the International Seminar in Family Planning in the Public Health Systems of Socialist Countries, Rostock, German Democratic Republic, October 1971.
213. Stampar, D. Croatia: Outcome of pregnancy in women whose requests for legal abortion have been denied. *Studies in Family Planning*, 1973, 4, 267-69.
214. Stoimenov, G., Neshkov, N., and Vasilev, D. Repercussions of legal restrictions for pregnancy interruption on birth rates. (In Bulgarian with English summary) *Akusherstvo i Ginekologiya*, 1972, 11, 1-7.
215. Stycos, J.M. Social class and preferred family size in Peru. In J.M. Stycos, *Human fertility in Latin America.* Ithaca, N.Y.: Cornell University Press, 1968, pp. 147-61.
216. Sun, T.H. Induced abortion in Taiwan. Unpublished paper, November 1970.
217. Sun, T.H., and Lee, C.H. Birth control experience in Taiwan. *Contraception*, 1971, 3, 241-60.
218. Svala, G. Sweden. *Country Profiles*, July 1972.

219. Sweden, Government of. Crown order No. 354 of 10 May 1963, Law No. 213 of 5 June 1963, Law No. 172 of 20 March 1964. *International Digest of Health Legislation*, 1966, 17, 152.
220. Sweezy, A.R. Recent light on the relation between socio-economic development and fertility decline. Paper prepared for Caltech-American Universities Fieldstaff Meeting, August1972.
221. Szabady, E., and Klinger, A. Pilot surveys of repeated abortion-seeking. *International Mental Health Research Newsletter*, 1972, 14, 6-9.
222. Tabah, L., and Samuel, R. Preliminary findings of a survey on fertility and attitudes toward family formation in Santiago, Chile. In C.V. Kiser (ed.), *Research in family planning.* Princeton, N.J.: Princeton University Press, 1962, pp. 263-304.
223. Taeuber, I.B. Chinese populations in transition: The city-states. *Population Index*, 1972, 38, 3-34.
224. Teitelbaum, M.S. International experience with fertility at or near replacement level. In C.F. Westoff and R. Parke, Jr. (eds.), *Demographic and social aspects of population growth.* Vol. 1 of the Commission on Population Growth and the American Future Research Reports. Washington: U.S. Government Printing Office, 1972, pp. 646-58.
225. Tietze, C. The demographic significance of legal abortion in Eastern Europe. *Demography*, 1964, 1, 119-25.
226. Tietze, C. Abortion laws and abortion practices in Europe. In A.J. Sobrero and C. McKee (eds.), *Advances in planned parenthood.* Vol. 5. Amsterdam: Excerpta Medica, International Congress Series No. 207, 1970, pp. 194-212.
227. Tietze, C. Abortion on request: Its consequences for population trends and public health. In R.B. Sloane (ed.), Psychiatric aspects of abortion. *Seminars in Psychiatry*, 1970, 2, 375-81.
228. Tietze, C. The potential impact of legal abortions on population growth in the United States. In C.F. Westoff and R. Parke, Jr. (eds.), *Demographic and social aspects of population growth.* Vol. 1 of the Commission on Population Growth and the American Future Research Reports. Washington: U.S. Government Printing Office, 1972, pp. 579-85.
229. Tietze, C. Two years' experience with a liberal abortion law: Its impact on fertility trends in New York City. *Family Planning Perspectives*, 1973, 5, 36-41.
230. Tietze, C. Personal communication, January 22, 1974.
231. Tietze, C., and Dawson, D. Induced abortion: A factbook. *Reports on Population/Family Planning*, December 1973, No. 14.
232. Tietze, C., and Lewit, S. Abortion. *Scientific American*, 1969, 220, 21-27.
233. Treffers, P.E. Role of induced abortion in the changing pattern of birth control in The Netherlands. (In Dutch with English summary) *Nederlands Tijdschrift voor Geneeskunde*, 1972, 116, 1459-66.

234. Tunisia, Government of. Décret-loi No. 73-2 du 26 Septembre 1973, portant modification de l'article 214 du Code Penal.
235. United Kingdom. *1967 abortion act: Comments and advice.* London: Medical Protection Society Ltd., undated.
236. United Kingdom, Office of Health Economics. *Family planning in Britain.* London: Her Majesty's Stationery Office, 1972.
237. United Kingdom, Office of Population Censuses and Surveys. *The Registrar General's statistical review of England and Wales. Part II, 1941-1971.* London: Her Majesty's Stationery Office, 1973.
238. United Kingdom, Office of Population Censuses and Surveys. *The Registrar General's statistical review of England and Wales for the year 1971: Supplement on abortion.* London: Her Majesty's Stationery Office, 1973.
239. United Nations, Department of Economic and Social Affairs, Statistical Office. *Population and vital statistics report: Data available as of 1 October 1973.* New York: Author, Statistical Papers, Series A, 25 (3-4), 1973.
240. United Nations, Statistical Office. *Demographic yearbooks.* New York: Author, various years.
241. United Nations, Statistical Office. Replies to supplementary questionnaire on legally induced abortion; various years. Unpublished.
242. United States Agency for International Development, Office of Population. *Population program assistance.* Washington: U.S. Government Printing Office, 1972.
243. United States Commission on Population Growth and the American Future. *Population and the American future: The report of the Commission on Population Growth and the American Future.* New York: New American Library (Signet), 1972 (unofficial advance version).
244. United States Department of Commerce, Bureau of the Census. Birth expectations and fertility, June 1972. *Current Population Reports*, April 1973, Series P-20, No. 248.
245. United States Department of Commerce, Bureau of the Census. Birth expectations of American wives, June 1973. *Current Population Reports*, June 1973, Series P-20, No. 254.
246. United States Department of Commerce, Bureau of the Census. Marital status and living arrangements March 1973. *Current Population Reports*, November 1973, Series P-20, No. 255.
247. United States Department of Health, Education, and Welfare, National Center for Health Statistics. Provisional statistics: Births, deaths, marriages, and divorces: Annual summary for the United States. *Monthly Vital Statistics Report*, issued annually.
248. United States Department of Health, Education, and Welfare, National Center for Health Statistics. Interval between first marriage and legitimate first birth, United States, 1964-1966. *Monthly Vital Statistics Report*, 1970, 18(12) (supplement); and *National Statistics Analysis: United States, 1965-1967*, May 1970, No. 1000, Series 21, No. 19.

249. United States Department of Health, Education, and Welfare, National Center for Health Statistics. Births, marriages, divorces, and deaths for June 1973. *Monthly Vital Statistics Report*, 1973, 22(6).
250. United States Department of Health, Education, and Welfare, National Center for Health Statistics. Summary report: Final natality statistics, 1969. *Monthly Vital Statistics Report*, 1973, 22(7) (supplement).
251. United States Supreme Court. *Roe vs. Wade (70-18) and Doe vs. Bolton (70-40).* Washington: Reporter of Decisions, syllabus, January 22, 1973.
252. Uruguay, Government of. Penal Code, Arts, 325-28, 24 January 1938. Cited in J.B. Carballa (ed.), *Penal Code* (2nd ed.). (In Spanish) Montevideo: Law Students Center, 1968.
253. Valaoras, V. The epidemiology of abortion in Greece. Paper presented at the International Planned Parenthood Federation Sixth Conference of the European and Near East Region, Budapest, September 1969.
254. Venkatacharya, K. Reduction in fertility due to induced abortion: A simulation model. *Demography*, 1972, 3, 339-52.
255. Viel, B. *The social consequences of population growth.* Washington: The Population Reference Bureau, 1969.
256. Viel, B. Abortion in Latin America in historical perspective. In H.P. David and S. Cambiaso (eds.), *Abortion and family planning practices in Latin America.* Washington: Pan American Health Organization, 1974, forthcoming.
257. Wagatsuma, T. The abortion program in Japan. *Journal of Reproductive Medicine*, 1971, 7(1), 16-19.
258. Wagner, M.M., and Wagner, M.G. Helping mothers in Denmark: Over two centuries of experience. Unpublished paper, Copenhagen, 1973.
259. Waisanen, F.B., and Durlak, J.T. A survey related to Costa Rican population dynamics. Paper presented at the American International Association for Economic and Social Development Meeting, San Jose, Costa Rica, 1966.
260. *The Washington Post.* Poverty, budget cuts spell Indian failure in birth control. September 15, 1973.
261. Washington, State of. Crimes and punishments: Chapter 9.02 on abortion. November 1970.
262. Watson, W.B. *1971 fertility-abortion survey: Quick report No. 16.* Seoul: The Population Council, 1971.
263. Watson, W.B. *1973 Korean Institute for Family Planning multipurpose survey: Quick report No. 17.* Seoul: The Population Council, 1973.
264. Watson, W.B., and Worth, G. Korea. *Studies in Family Planning*, 1972, 3, 132-35.
265. Weller, R.H., Macisco, J.J., Jr., and Martine, G.R. The relative importance of the components of urban growth in Latin America. *Demography*, 1971, 8, 225-32.

266. Westoff, C.F. The modernization of U.S. contraceptive practice. *Family Planning Perspectives*, 1972, 3(3), 9-12.

267. Woolf, M. *Family intentions: An enquiry undertaken for the General Registrar's Office.* London: Office of Population Censuses and Surveys, Her Majesty's Stationery Office, 1971.

268. World Health Organization. *Spontaneous and induced abortion: Report of a WHO scientific group.* Geneva, WHO Technical Report Series, No. 461, 1970.

269. Worth, G., Watson, W.B., Han, D.W., Finnigan, O.D., and Keeny, S.M. Korea/Taiwan 1970: Report on the national family planning programs. *Studies in Family Planning*, 1971, 2, 57-69.

270. Yen, C.H. Taiwan. *Studies in Family Planning*, 1973, 4, 118-23.

271. Yugoslavia, Government of. Decree No. 33 of 16 February 1960. *International Digest of Health Legislation*, 1961, 12, 619-22

272. Zarate, A.O. Differential fertility in Monterrey, Mexico: Prelude to transition? *Milbank Memorial Fund Quarterly*, 1967, 45(2), Part 1, 93-108.

273. Zelnik, M., and Kantner, J.F. Sexuality, contraception and pregnancy among young unwed females in the United States. In C.F. Westoff and R. Parke, Jr. (eds.), *Demographic and social aspects of population growth.* Vol. 1 of the Commission on Population Growth and the American Future Research Reports. Washington: U.S. Government Printing Office, 1972, pp. 355-74.

274. Zetterberg, H. Unpublished communication of the Swedish Institute of Opinion Formation, Stockholm, 1967.

About the Author

Jean van der Tak is a Research Associate for the Transnational Family Research Institute, affiliated with the American Institutes for Research, Washington, D.C. She received the M.A. in demography in 1970 from the Center for Population Research, The Joseph and Rose Kennedy Institute for the Study of Human Reproduction and Bioethics, Georgetown University, where she was a Research Associate from 1971 to 1973. She has also been a Research Associate for the Netherlands Interuniversity Demographic Institute, The Hague; and a Research Assistant for the Population Crisis Committee, Washington, D.C. Ms. van der Tak has contributed to *Population Studies*, and the *American Journal of Public Health.*